DARE TO BE VITAL

D1739064

DARE TO BE VITAL

*Your Blueprint For
A Vibrant Life*

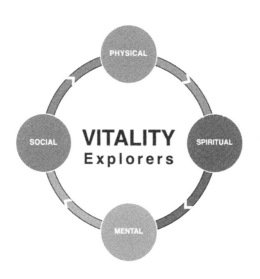

Allan Mishra, MD

TABLE OF CONTENTS

DARE TO BE VITAL

PRAISE FOR THE FIRST EDITION

"Great book with practical and simple steps to improve today. Don't wait; get, read, and start applying these lessons now!"

"Really enjoyed this read. It's never easy trying to codify a complex message but Dr. Mishra does so exceedingly well."

"Dr. Mishra distills research and insights from a variety of disciplines into easily understood summaries, brings them to life with personal experience that is emotionally relatable and gives the reader a simple but powerful action planning toolkit."

"I loved the Vitality Essentials course book. It was a thoughtful guide to getting your priorities in order for life and what makes life important. I like the interactive portions of each chapter that force you to make vital changes or at least think about them."

"Dr. Mishra adds an honest and useful guide for living a more fulfilling life. His education and career have placed him on the front lines of observing the personal attributes that allow some individuals to achieve optimal meaning and satisfaction in their lives — what the author calls 'vitality'."

"The beauty and thrust of Dr. Mishra's vitality mantra is an active, individualized accounting of some real core and digestible concepts."

PREFACE TO SECOND EDITION

I f your future self could talk to your present self, what advice would it give?

Your future self would tell you you're in control of your circumstances. It would advise you to take ownership of your decisions and choices. It would recommend that you complain less and do more.

But you are living in the present. You don't have a crystal ball into the future. That doesn't mean you can't act today to influence your tomorrow.

This second edition of *Dare To Be Vital* represents a complete revision. It is my attempt to enhance the value of the book for readers.

Three more years of exploring how to lead a vital life are embedded in this edition. It includes the work I do to teach my ENERGIZE Your Life course for Stanford Continuing Studies.

This edition also draws upon my work producing *Vitality Explorer News*. This is a publication on Substack dedicated to enhancing global vitality, one person at a time. Each week we review several scientific articles and then apply that vetted information to our daily lives. This can be found at: https:// vitalityexplorers.substack.com/. Interested readers can also join VitalityExplorers.com for free. This is a community of people dedicated to helping each other enhance vitality.

Finally, this new version takes advantage of being able to share my ideas about vitality with elite organizations such as Stanford University, the University of Cambridge, the University of Michigan, Google, Apple and many others. My job presenting to these audiences has been to teach people how to lead an optimal life. More often, it has been me that has learned many crucial lessons from my audiences. This new version shares many of those lessons and stories.

It has been an honor and a blessing to explore vitality scientifically for more than seven years. My goal continues to be:

Enhance Global Vitality, One Person at a Time.

Allan Mishra, MD
February 2023

INTRODUCTION

Think of yourself as a savvy investor in your own life. How should you allocate your time, talent and treasure to live your best possible life? That's what this book offers. It is designed to give you specific actionable ways to enhance your vitality. Let's begin by telling you the story of how I became a vitality explorer.

The Search for Vitality

Waves from the Great Barrier Reef splashed at my naked feet. I was running effortlessly southbound on Four Mile Beach in northern Australia. The sand was firm but not hard and warm but not hot. After about two miles, I stopped, stretched, and swam into the idyllic Coral Sea for about 10 minutes. I then ran northbound along the same stretch of beach toward a spectacular eight-story-tall palm tree.

As I ran, I did a system check. Did my back hurt? No. Did my legs hurt? No. Was I short of breath? No. I galloped with a confidence I hadn't experienced in years. Did my head hurt? No. Was I worried about anything at that moment? No.

In a word, I felt vital.

We often dwell on times of trial and try to figure out what went wrong. I paused at that moment in time to contemplate why everything seemed so right. I felt spectacular and wanted to understand why. Physically, I was strong. I was able to run and swim quickly and without pain. Mentally, my head was clear and I felt calm. Socially, I was in harmony with my friends and family. Spiritually, I felt close to God and also believed I had found my purpose for being on the planet. I wasn't just living well that day. I was living somewhere beyond well.

Finding an actionable biomarker for vitality became my new scientific quest when I returned from my trip to Australia.

I wanted to figure out how to live as vitally as possible and share my findings with as many people as possible. I wanted to drink from the Holy Grail of vitality.

While I expected my vitality to be closely correlated to how much sleep I got or how well I had eaten, I was stunned to find a whole other set of correlates that no DNA test, blood test, or heart monitor could decipher. My mental, social, and spiritual well-being had to be equally in balance with my physical well-being for me to be optimal. I could've gotten eight hours of sleep and eaten less than 1800 calories in a day and still felt less than vital for the day if I was feeling angry, lonely, anxious, etc. The same was true if my spiritual, social, or work lives were difficult. It turned out that these non-physical parameters dramatically affected my ability to sleep and work out. The concept of vitality as being linked to the interdependence of my physical, mental, social, and spiritual wellness crystallized in my mind.

Putting Vitality Into Practice

I started writing down my ideas and formulated a series of diagrams. Through these exercises I returned to the "A-Ha!" moment I had earlier. While vitality can't be measured by biologic assessments, it can be assessed by your overall quality of life.

Vitality is about a balance of physical, mental, social, and spiritual well-being. I started to get clarity on how these four pillars broke down into eight essential building blocks of vitality:

- Time
- Discipline
- Purpose
- Sleep
- Fitness
- Closeness
- Service
- Hope

For good physical health we must sleep well and focus on our fitness, which includes diet and exercise. For good mental health, we must have hope and be disciplined. For good social health, we must focus on developing closeness with our friends and family and seek to serve others whenever possible. For good spiritual health, we must precisely define our purpose and manage our time accordingly. The pairings were fundamentally interrelated. And, at the same time, each individual building block also is ultimately interrelated with every other one. And since genetic markers are not directly related to vitality, you don't have to be born with any of these skills. It's possible for anyone regardless of age or physical condition to be vital.

After this series of realizations, I started talking about vitality with my patients, friends, and family. I spoke to them about how if you sleep better, you can exercise more. Exercising helps you manage your weight and also reduces your stress. Having a specific goal or purpose helps focus your efforts and provides hope for the future. And I explained how each of these building blocks was actually a skill that could be acquired with practice.

Later, I realized my chosen profession contained a perfect metaphor for vitality. Orthopedic surgeons focus on treating injuries of ligaments, tendons, bones, and other forms of connective tissue. Remember the song you learned as a child: "The toe bone is connected to the foot bone. The foot bone is connected to the ankle bone. "? Since then, you probably learned that it's true: Most of us discover through injuries or aging bodies that if our toe bone isn't working, we can't run well. A bad toe adversely affects the function of the knee. A bad toe can alter the biomechanics of your hip, which is connected to your spine. And on and on.

Vitality works similarly to the human skeleton, even though the "bones" are different. Instead, Time, Discipline, Purpose, Sleep Fitness, Closeness, Service and Hope make up the skeleton of vitality. Together these "bones" form an octagon of skills that can be learned. And one of these skills alone can help strengthen or weaken the others.

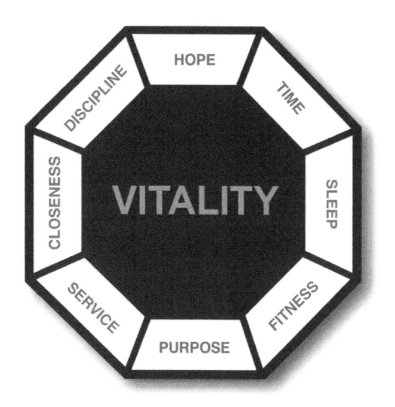

The Vitality Octagon

If we don't define our purpose precisely, we lose hope.
Without hope it is impossible to be disciplined. Without discipline, we will not be able to keep up an exercise routine,
and so on. Vitality is the byproduct of optimizing these eight
skills. And by stockpiling each of these skills, we invest in

an insurance policy for not just our current vitality but our future vitality as well.

Together these skills work to strengthen the four pillars of vitality: Physical, Mental, Social, and Spiritual Health. Consider the pillars as overarching categories of vitality supported by the skills within the octagon.

I used to think of the pillars as static and represented them with this image:

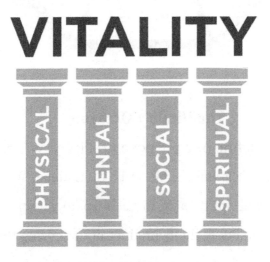

After scientifically studying vitality for seven years, I now understand vitality is a process, not a state of being. I now think of it more like a flywheel. Each pillar of vitality is connected to the others helping enhance or inhibit it. Our physical and mental wellness are intimately connected. We are mentally sharper when we are physically in better shape. Our spiritual and social wellness are also predictive of our mental and physical wellness. Too often we ignore these interconnections. We fail to recognize the power that is inherent in the vitality flywheel. (See image below)

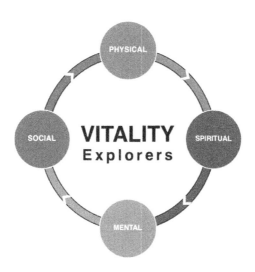

The Vitality Flywheel

We need to realize our vitality is a personal journey, not a destination. Vital people seek to continually improve themselves. Your vitality is also not carved in stone by your genes, financial situation, or social status. It can be modified and elevated by the choices you make.

You can learn how to be vital. I want to help you find your highest level of vitality. I want to help you master each of the parameters within the Vitality Octagon and live your best possible life.

Now, we can talk about vitality until we're blue in the face. However, only <u>you</u> can choose to be vital. There is no waiting or hoping to be vital. Stop bingeing at the buffet of excuses and take ownership over your vitality today. Set an intention to enhance your vitality. Challenge yourself to become your most vital self. Consider the rest of this book as your personal vitality manual. Don't simply read the book. Study it and complete the exercises within each lesson.

I'll be your guide, coach, and cheerleader with one specific mantra:

Dare To Be Vital.

THINK WITH TIME IN MIND

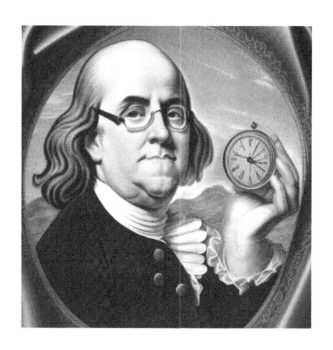

"Lost time is never found."

Benjamin Franklin

H ow do we arrest the time bandits that run our lives? It's both easy and difficult.

A shiny crimson card was waiting for me when I returned from a vacation for my 50th birthday. I had to Google "AARP" to confirm the acronym stood for "American Association of Retired Persons." Did this new piece of bloody-colored plastic mean I could now retire? Or, did it simply confirm I am officially old and beyond the desirable 18-49 demographic?

I picked a number out of the air and said to myself, I'll live to 85 years old. That would mean I have about 35 years left. That also is 12,775 days, 306,600 hours, 18 million minutes, or about 1.1 billion seconds. It turns out the Social Security Actuarial Life Table pegged my remaining time at 29.45 more years. That is about 928 million seconds. I averaged the two numbers and came up with about one billion seconds left on the planet for me to live.

To sharpen my focus, I started measuring how I spent my seconds. Each 1000 seconds equals about 17 minutes. What did I do with my last 1000 seconds? Was it a wise use of my time? Each 10,000 seconds equals about three hours. Would I later be happy with how I spent those 10,000 seconds? Simply measuring how you spend your seconds, much like calorie counting, will alter your behavior.

Then I asked myself a crucial question: How would I change my life if every second were precious?

Would I stop wasting time being angry about the situations I cannot control?

Would I seek to better understand the purpose for every interaction in life?

Would I treat every person I encounter as an important human being?

Million Second Challenge

Perhaps you have more or less seconds left in your life than me. You may be in your 20s, 40s, 60s or 80s. One thing is true at any age. *All seconds are important.* We should consider them precious like a luxury watch or diamond bracelet.

Think about how to best spend your next one million seconds. This is about 12 days. Look at a calendar and circle the date, 12 days from now.

Now, begin to think with time in mind and write down how you hope to best spend your next one million seconds. How can you enhance your vitality by using your time optimally?

I call this the *Million Second Challenge.*

Do your future self a favor and write down several specific ideas on piece of paper or in a journal. Think of yourself like a reporter. Write a headline that will be published one million seconds from now.

Writing down your future headlines is an excellent way to plan how to spend your most precious non-renewable resource. Your final headline -- the one you want to have at your funeral -- is the most difficult, but also the most important, one to consider. Think about that but focus now on the next million seconds.

Having a headline in mind helps me refine the list of what I must do to make it come true. Start by writing tomorrow's headline. Here are a few possibilities:

- "My day was awesome."
- "Today I made a difference for at least one person."
- "Today, I bet on myself and worked toward my goals."
- "Hit the gym, ate well and lost a pound."
- "Connected with my old friend from college on the phone."

Think about the end of your day. How can your actions during the day make a positive difference?

If you think you deserve more money in your present job and you want a raise, today should be the day to ask for it. Or, will today be the day you quit your job and seek a better one?

That is thinking with a day in mind. What if you could think past tomorrow? Expand your headline to a week. What would those headlines look like?

- "This week, I lost two pounds."
- "I checked in with three old friends this week."
- "I eliminated all distractions and finished my term paper early."

By writing a headline in advance, you force yourself to think about how you're going to accomplish that headline. The *Million Second Challenge* headline should be something you can do in the next 12 days. This is a time horizon that we can see. That makes it easier for us to think about it. Our future selves become blurry when we think too far into the future.

Pause for a moment and write down two things you could do in the next million seconds. Keep the entries tight and specific.

Now, let's move on to a longer horizon and think about six months from now. What could you do in that time frame? Here are some possibilities:

- "My knees feel great because I finally lost 20 pounds."
- "My relationship with my daughter is stellar because I made time to have dinner with her almost every night."
- "Volunteering at the Boys and Girls Club once a week dramatically enhanced my vitality."

Let's now extend the time frame to a year. What would a headline look like for you in 12 months? Don't try to limit yourself. Think boldly.

I'll share mine with you as I write this lesson:

"Vitality Explorers now has more than a million active participants each month."

That's what I hope will be a headline one year from now. Writing a headline about aiming to enhance the world's vitality at that scale is a little crazy. Am I bold or delusional? I am practicing prophetic thinking by writing such a headline for myself. I am thinking with time in mind. Thinking of that headline helps me avoid distractions such as too much streaming media and the relentless inane political banter on television that masquerades as news.

Think what you want your headlines to be for your life. Start practicing prophetic thinking today. Your future self will thank you.

Remember, thinking about how you spend your time is never a waste of time.

Here are thoughts to consider as you think about how to optimize your time:

Seek to live in the now. This means to always be present. Listen when someone is speaking to you. Put your phone down and look that person in the eyes. Just enjoy being in the present moment.

Avoid energy vampires. These are the people and activities that literally suck your blood and bone marrow. It is not possible to eliminate all contact with energy vampires because they could be your boss or maybe even a family member. But, limiting time spent with them is crucial.

Embrace energy angels. These are people and activities that enhance your vitality. Schedule time to be those people and activities that increase your energy.

The goal is to be ruthless with your precious time.

Many of us believe we have zero time to focus on our personal vitality. I reject this claim. I believe we are bingeing at the buffet of excuses. That is why the first exercise of *Vitality*

Essentials is to learn how to eliminate this horrible habit. Please take some time and execute on the exercises below. The goal of these exercises is to help you become an optimal manager of your precious time.

Exercise 1
Stop Bingeing at the Buffet of Excuses.

What are the top three reasons you do not focus on enhancing your vitality?

- Work or School Demands
- Lack of Sleep
- Financial Challenges
- Medical Issues
- Relationship Issues
- Childcare / Eldercare Responsibilities
- Commute Time
- Housework / Meal Preparation
- Lack of Access to Exercise Equipment
- Issues With Overeating, Drinking, or Substance Abuse
- Other:

Turn the reasons into barriers and list two specific ways to overcome the barriers.

1.

2.

Exercise 2
Efficient Ranking

List your top ten things to do in the next month. This could be things at home, things at work or things in your commu- nity. Be careful to rank order them with the most important ones in the top three.

1.

2.

3.

4.

5.

6.

7.

8.

9.

10.

Now, give yourself permission to focus 90% of your energy and enthusiasm on only the top three. And, give yourself permission to spend zero time on the bottom three.

Make sure you review and revise your to do list on a daily basis. Don't allow anything that doesn't absolutely matter to creep into the top three on that list.

Don't fret about not doing much to accomplish the bottom three. Remember, you put them at the bottom of the list for a reason.

Exercise 3

Write Your Future Headlines

Tomorrow:

One Week:

One Month:

One Year:

Final Headline (What you want to be said at your funeral):

Vital Time Story
The Shovel Next to the Grave

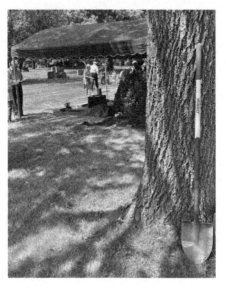

You never know when the shovel will be for you.

I went to a funeral after an unexpected death in the family in the summer of 2021. It was a terrible and also awesome weekend.

It was terrible because of the loss of a special life that made this world a better place. A life dedicated to the love and support of those in need.

It was awesome because I connected with a large portion of my family and many old friends.

The flight out during the Covid pandemic was occupied with petty thoughts of what is wrong in my life.

The flight back was filled with the joy of what is right in my life.

I travelled to support and love my family during a difficult time. I've unfortunately been to many funerals. My first was my mom's funeral. I was just nine. My last will be my own.

The shovel leaning against the tree next to the fresh grave site assaulted me.

- It screamed at me to forgive more and complain less.
- It asked me why I didn't think more of others and less of myself.
- It begged me to understand: You don't know when I am coming for you.

When will the shovel be for you or a loved one? We cannot know the future.

We can, however, seek to be the best possible version of ourselves while we wait for our time.

We can strive each day to help out those in need.

We can strive to find and execute on our peak purpose.

We can strive to solve the difficult problems facing our communities, our countries and the world.

Don't wait until tomorrow.

Don't wait until the shovel is for you.

Begin today to be a better version of yourself than yesterday.

LESSON TWO

DOUBLE DOWN ON DISCIPLINE

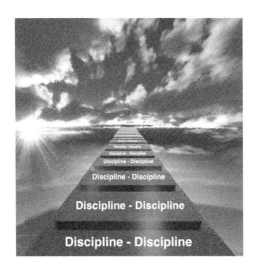

"It's not the Mountain we Conquer but Ourselves"

Sir Edmund Hilary

We discussed how we must be disciplined with our precious time in the last chapter. Now, we will learn how to double down on discipline. This analogy is related to the concept of doubling your bet when you have the excellent starting hand of eleven in a game of blackjack. Doubling down means to increase your commitment.

Discipline is the ability to control how you live, work or behave. It is often associated with physical or mental training. It can also be connected to a specific code of conduct.

Seneca the ancient Roman Stoic philosopher implored us to seek discomfort to toughen ourselves. I suggest we follow his example and tone our toughness with discipline.

This is not easy. It reminds me of an axiom I learned during my orthopedic surgery residency. A wise doctor taught me if you cannot figure out the right thing to do, it is usually the more difficult option. He suggested I develop the discipline to always choose the harder path if I wasn't sure. This is some of the best advice I have ever received.

I've unlocked the right answer for countless patients by following my mentor's advice. I realize the best pathway is the more difficult one. I sulk for a moment and then get on with the challenging business of identifying the appropriate next step knowing it will be difficult.

I review a checklist I was taught in my first year of medical school to approach the problem from a systems perspective. I begin with the worst-case scenarios such as severe infection, a blood vessel injury, or cancer. I carefully rule in or out the options using the patient's history, physical exam and test results. Having the discipline to go over every possibility calms me down in the middle of a storm.

We aren't wasting time and effort by being disciplined or choosing the harder path. We are simply choosing the best long-term option. Doing so helps us save time. It also helps unlock meaningful solutions.

It is crucial to demand more discipline from ourselves than anyone else. When we know we have done our best, others recognize the effort even if we fail in the short term. We serve as an example to other people when we consistently make disciplined choices. Doing our best when the road is rocky also allows us to forgive ourselves if the outcome is not ideal.

Demanding excellence from yourself can only come from within. It is not something someone can give you. Not choosing to double down on discipline has consequences. Not being disciplined comes with a steep price. The bill is not immediately due. It arrives later in the form of consequences. Most of them are minor. Some are major. One of the worst consequences is knowing we have not done our best.

I've learned the lesson of doubling down on discipline many times during my career as an orthopedic surgeon and sports medicine specialist. I also learned it from former Secretary of State Condoleezza Rice.

"It is a privilege to struggle," according to Dr. Rice. She grew up in racially segregated Birmingham, Alabama, in the 1960s. She went on to become the first African American

Secretary of State and Provost of Stanford University. Her name is derived from the musical term, *con dolcezza,* which means "with sweetness" in Italian. Ironically, she has had to deal with significant bitterness in her life. She has had to overcome many obstacles during her stellar career.

I had the honor of being a speaker at Stanford University during the Campbell Trophy Summit with Dr. Rice. The summit honors elite college football players for their academics, football excellence and community service. She talked about how she had to work hard to be twice as good in order to overcome the many obstacles in her life. She embodies courage which is acting in the face of fear. She also discussed the power of embracing pain as a pathway to change. Enduring consistent pain requires epic discipline. And epic discipline fosters toughness which is the ability to struggle, survive and thrive.

Dr. Rice convinced her audience it is a privilege to struggle. Her example helps us understand why we should embrace adversity instead of trying to avoid it. Next time you face adversity or challenge, think of it as an opportunity for post traumatic growth. This unique type of growth is often under recognized. We have all heard of post traumatic pain but rarely realize the value of pain. It can help you make better choices. It can help motivate you to get a better job or relationship. Don't discount its value. Your resilience and toughness rise from overcoming the stress and strain of adversity, not from whining about it or trying to avoid it.

Adversity strikes everyone. Sometimes it hits like lightning and ignites a raging fire. That happened to me when I was nine. My mom died of a brain tumor after suffering for five months in the hospital and enduring several operations.

I spiraled into an abyss and was saved by my fifth-grade teacher. He caught me smoking in the restroom at school with a couple of juvenile delinquents. The guys that lured me into smoking went directly to the principal's office. My fifth-grade teacher had me stand against the wall and he looked me directly in my tearful eyes. He told me to stop feeling sorry for myself. He acknowledged the death of my beloved saintly mother. He then told me he believed in me and that I had a bright future. He demanded I take responsibility for my actions. I was petrified he would tell my demanding father. He didn't. Instead, he ignited a fire in me that burns to this day to be a better person. To take responsibility for my actions. To honor my mother's memory with my best efforts. Mr. Paull literally changed my life.

I rarely share that story with anyone but was forced to at Google. My pastor nominated me to give a talk there about spirituality because of my vitality work. He didn't tell me until I had been accepted to speak. I presented my rough draft version of my speech to him a few days before the event on the Google campus. He liked it but thought I needed to share my story about being confronted by my fifth-grade teacher after my mother died. I recoiled in horror with that suggestion.

I didn't want to be vulnerable especially at Google. I have lived in the Silicon Valley for more than two decades with my gilded mask of perfection tightly secured around my face. I reluctantly agreed to share my childhood challenges. It wasn't easy but it was freeing. I could finally admit that I am still scarred by losing my mother at such a young age. I could admit I don't have it all figured out. I could admit I still miss my mom.

I share the story of my mom because I know all of us have had to endure challenges in our lives. I buried my history of childhood trauma for most of my life. I refused to confront how it forever changed me. Only once I began to open up to people about it did I begin to understand how surviving it made me stronger. Each of you reading this book has a difficulty that has shaped you.

Adversity comes in many forms---physical, mental, social, and spiritual. Each form of adversity requires a different type of discipline and toughness to survive. I believe each of us is blessed with innate ability to combat adversity. We have the power to survive epic challenges. But where does this power come from? It comes from within. We need, however, to learn how to cultivate and strengthen it. We also need to learn how to summon discipline on demand.

Discipline is a cousin of toughness. We toughen our minds and bodies when we are disciplined. And, toughness is a vitality skill that rises from the ashes of surviving raging fires. It doesn't come from acting like snowplows that push away all forms of adversity. Toughness doesn't come from acting like a victim. It also doesn't come from trying to avoid pain. It comes from metabolizing pain into meaningful action.

Discipline is like muscle. Muscles enlarge in response to load. Lift weights consistently and you will see a response in your muscle tone. Muscles also release powerful molecules called myokines when we contract them. These molecules not only stimulate our muscles but also improve the function of our hearts and brains.

Similarly, discipline improves many parts of our lives. It helps us organize our time. It helps us make better choices. Our ability to be disciplined also rises when we practice navigating difficult pathways. It rises when we realize most severe pain is transient. It rises when we learn to live with some pain as the cost of being alive. It rises when we practice being consistent with our work to improve our physical, mental, social and spiritual well-being.

An excellent way to enhance our discipline is follow Seneca's advice and seek discomfort. Embrace being uncomfortable. Doing so makes us appreciate even more the times in our lives when we are not in pain.

We should also seek to optimize our toughness. Vital toughness is the product of having a prepared body, mind, and soul. Toughness is the ability to absorb energy like a punch and not break. It requires a combination of strength and flexibility. Terminator toughness only exists in those individuals who have survived the epic stress of a crucible.

So, begin today to double down on discipline. Your future self will thank you.

Exercise 4

List two times when you struggled significantly in your life:

1.

2.

Now, describe how you grew from those times.
What did you learn? List two specific things.

1

2.

We can learn more about discipline and toughness from the following two stories.

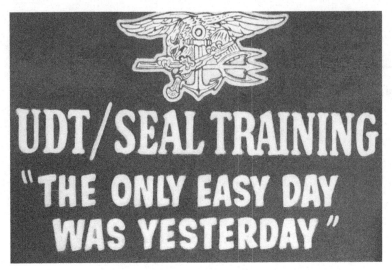

"The Only Easy Day Was Yesterday"

The yard looks like something many of us may have seen at our elementary schools during recess. It is a large square blacktop area ringed by chin-up bars and several signs. Reaching back into my distant memory brings up a vision of playing kickball on this type of surface.

There were, however, several differences. Strangely shaped white markers adorned the black top in perfect rows. It was difficult to figure out what they represented from a distance. Standing close over the markers it was obvious they represented a pair of flippers.

Each set of stenciled flippers on the blacktop was for a Navy SEAL candidate. A blue sign next to the yard screamed out in yellow letters: "The only easy day was yesterday." A small bell with a thin string attached to it could also be found in the back corner of the workout yard.

The United States Navy's Sea, Air and Land Teams (SEALs) train in an isolated part of Coronado Island, California on this blacktop yard. All SEALs must complete basic underwater demolition / SEAL training. Part of that training is hell week where the instructors do their best to get candidates to quit. The training is known as some of the most rigorous in the world. No part of it is easy.

All training is voluntary. Any candidate can quit at any time. They must signal their desire to quit by ringing the bell in the workout yard three times. I've been honored to visit the SEAL training facility multiple times. I've seen the bell, the famous obstacle course and even witnessed candidates work on their hand-to-hand combat skills. It is a special and inspiring place. The SEAL team members have many say-ings. One of them is, "Don't Ring The Bell."

This means to never quit. Almost all of us will never have what it takes to become a SEAL. I think, however, we can learn from their epic discipline. We can learn from their ability to deal with pain and adversity.

"Embrace the suck."

That is another SEAL mantra. It means to figure out how to deal with the physical and mental pain associated with the training process. I've interviewed many SEALs and asked what it takes to become one. To a person, they talk about discipline. They saw many of their candidate mates fail during training because they were too soft. They were high maintenance like a fancy sports car. The ones that sur-vived the training were low maintenance four-wheel drive pick-up trucks. They never needed much and never quit. They fueled themselves with discipline. Discipline in train-ing. Discipline to endure physical and mental suffering.

Discipline to continue when their brains and bodies were beyond exhaustion.

We will never know exactly what it takes to become a Navy SEAL. We can, however, channel our inner SEAL and seek to be more like them. We can remind ourselves that yesterday was the only easy day. We can embrace the suck and try to never ring the bell.

We can also learn from Kara Lawson. She is the women's basketball coach at Duke University. She talks about not waiting for the easy bus.

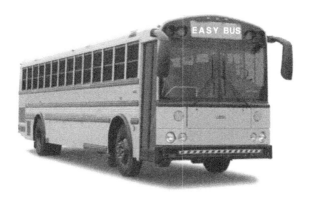

I understand the intrinsic value of hard work. I also value the ability to perform under pressure. Unfortunately, I find myself sometimes trying to hitch a ride on the easy bus. I think I want a life of leisure with boundless resources to do whatever I want whenever I want. No more struggles or feeling bad. I want to be on the glide path to the *Vitality Zone*.

I'm also sometimes allergic to adversity. I overreact to small problems thinking they are monumental. Then, I remember something crucial. Nothing I have ever done of lasting value personally or professionally was simple or easy. The journey to meaning in my life has always been difficult and demanded sacrifice.

That's why Coach Lawson's message to her team resonated with me. Here are some more of her platinum pieces of advice:

- "Don't get discouraged if it is hard. It is supposed to be."
- "You become someone that handles hard better."
- "It is a mental shift."

Her message is profound.

We need to stop waiting for the easy bus. She also implores her team to "make yourself a person that handles hard well and you're going to be great." She believes meaningful pur- suits in life go to people who embrace difficulty.

I think hard work has intrinsic value. We feel better about ourselves when we execute on something difficult with dis- cipline. Our confidence rises. Our self-esteem and mental health improve. And, your vitality soars.

Exercise 5

Struggle and suffering are parts of life. A strange but crucial question for vital people is:

What are you willing to suffer for?

List two things below:

1.

2.

PINPOINT YOUR PEAK PURPOSE

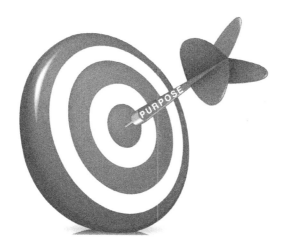

"Get Busy Living or Get Busy Dying."

The Shawshank Redemption

A s I began exploring vitality, I realized I needed a way to characterize how we live. I discovered through trial, error, and exhaustive research several zones of living. I call them the *Four Zones of Living*.

Many, if not most of us, are living in what I call *The Surviving Zone*: we are physically and mentally healthy but know there's something missing; we are on autopilot, more-or-less surviving rather than thriving. Others are in *The Sliding Zone*, beginning to break down in some significant way, whether physically, mentally, socially, or spiritually. Even worse are those in *The Burnout Zone*, falling into substance abuse or making terrible personal choices.

The Four Zones of Living

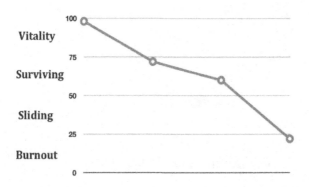

Falling into the Burnout Zone

Those of us in *The Surviving Zone* are functional but not vital. Ignoring concerns that arise in this zone leads to slipping into *The Sliding Zone. The Sliding Zone* is dangerous, like standing on the edge of a cliff near the ocean. The soil is unstable. There are loose rocks under your feet. A stiff breeze, a subtle misstep, or a small push and you'll head over the cliff. You can still, however, back away from the cliff. You can choose to move to safer ground. But you need to act.

Once we hit *The Sliding Zone,* we often fail to execute at work, home, or school. We miss deadlines. Or, we make poor time choices. We fail to prioritize sleep, exercise, or friendships. We claim our incessant work is to provide for our families. Ironically, we never make time for them. We snap at people we love. Our sleep suffers. Our friendships wither. We neglect our physical fitness. We gain 10 pounds. We try to numb ourselves with alcohol, food, or more powerful substances. A frenetic pace coupled with anger and profound fatigue replaces any sense of strength or contentment.

At the bottom of the cliff is *The Burnout Zone*. This is where waves are crashing with increasing intensity. The water is cold. Darkness envelops you. You feel alone and helpless. You catastrophize any problem in your life. Occasionally, it is possible to climb out of *The Burnout Zone* without assistance. Most often, however, getting out of *The Burnout Zone* requires help.

Unfortunately, burnout is at epidemic levels in our society today. There are myriad causes. Our work can be a primary source of burnout. High professional fulfillment is rare. The culprits may be arrogant managers, no control of one's work schedule, and/or inadequate sleep. A mismatch of your purpose and the organization's mission also can fuel burnout. And we often ignore our most important relationships until they are severely damaged. When you stop making time to listen, understand, and appreciate your friends and family, you risk falling into contempt and relationship burnout.

Then there's *The Vitality Zone*. This is where you are living your best life in a purposeful, energetic, and engaged manner. The good news is you can make the decision to be more vital, no matter what zone you are currently in. So, what can you do to increase your chances of living vitally?

Rising into the Vitality Zone

Defining your purpose is the crucial primary step on your journey into *The Vitality Zone*. Purpose can be defined as an aspiration or a desire to achieve something. Purpose can also spark hope. We will discuss service and hope more in our last lesson.

In June 2020, just as the COVID pandemic was beginning to rage I was asked to host a vitality webinar for the greater Stanford community on Zoom. The first task was to assess the audience's vitality and determine what needs they had. I asked the participants to rate themselves on the vitality octagon parameters. Surprisingly, I found a substantial correlation between having a high sense of purpose and having a high sense of hope.

This helped me with the webinar and my vitality work. I'm not sure how to teach someone how to enhance their sense of hope. My data suggests, however, that if I can improve their sense of purpose, their hope will rise. The rest of this lesson and the next one focus on helping us understand the value of purpose and how to identify our professional and personal purposes.

Scientific data has shown purpose can be a self-sustaining source of motivation. It can function as an excellent time management tool and improves mental well-being. It also provides structure to our lives. Importantly, having an elevated sense of purpose is associated with lower mortality and less risk of chronic disease. That is why purpose is a foundational component of vitality.

Purpose can be transformative, or it can be destructive. It will kill your vitality if you hate your purpose. Your vitality will rise if you identify a meaningful purpose.

Remember how vitality is similar to your skeleton? Your purpose is like your spine. It is your foundation. You suffer pain if your spine is weak or out of alignment. You will never be vital without a strong, guiding purpose.

Your present purpose is easy to define. It is a function of how you spend your time and energy. Your aspirational purpose is how you hope to spend your time and energy. Purpose can also be defined as your rationale for living. It is your personal answer to the question of why you are here on this planet.

There is a hierarchy of purpose that starts with defining short-term goals. A short-term goal could be: I want to run a 10-kilometer race. Or, I want to find a new job. Or, I'm going to volunteer at a homeless shelter. The hierarchy then progresses to executing on a prioritized set of goals. This is when you have a list of goals and sort those goals based on a long-term life mission. This is close to the apex of purpose. Finding your true calling is the mountaintop of purpose. I call this your peak purpose. A peak purpose is like love. You will know it when you find it. It may also take a lifetime.

Once you define your purpose, it becomes your life's GPS. It helps guide and direct your hourly, daily, weekly, and monthly decisions. It also helps you say no to projects and people that don't fit into your purpose. It is the rock upon which you build your vitality. It is also your most valuable modifiable vitality asset.

Your Purpose Today

I struggled for years trying to identify my peak purpose. I wasn't spending my time as wisely as possible. Interestingly, I also discovered when I was spending my time on something that was important to me, I brought more energy to the task.

A powerful way to figure out your purpose is to ask yourself a difficult question.

What are you willing to suffer for?

Muhammad Ali hated to train. He knew, however, that if he pushed himself to suffer during training that he had a better chance to win in his next boxing match. Here is a quote from him to consider as you contemplate what your peak purpose could be:

"Suffer now and live the rest of your life as a champion."

To help you define your current purpose, record how you spend your time during the upcoming week in the chart below. Then rate how much energy you bring to each moment.

Exercise 6
Purpose Identification Template

Day	Activity	Time	Energy (0-10)
Sun			
Mon			
Tues			
Wed			
Thurs			
Fri			
Sat			

Think what you care about most in this life. What brings you joy? What puts a smile on your face? Incorporate that into your purpose. Life is amazing but we never know when we will have our last best day. It is therefore crucial to have some fun.

We can also have a professional and a personal purpose. These purposes can evolve or even radically change with time. Let's learn from a professional purpose expert.

My close friend Dave is a successful business executive. He has held several CEO positions during his illustrious career. Prior to becoming a CEO, he was charged with turning around a division in a company that was struggling. The division sold soap and surgical drapes to hospitals. Their products were excellent but sales were lagging. It was Dave's job to rally the team and drive sales.

He hosted a weekend retreat and discussed the purpose behind their products. He understood it must have been difficult for the team to be proud of selling their products based only on their functional value. That was indeed true. Dave reviewed the internal company data proving their products reduced the risk of deadly hospital-acquired infections. That's when he had his purpose "epiphany."

He told the sales team they were not selling soap and sheets. They were saving lives. That simple but profound purpose shift increased sales by 20%. Saving lives with superior products became the purpose of the division. He changed their tagline to: "Cleaner, Safer, Healthier."

Dave's redefinition of the organization's purpose was transformative. He is a savant about helping companies perfect their professional purpose. He has done it many times with a wide variety of companies.

Pause and contemplate what the optimal purpose could be for your business. Higher profitability and employee satisfaction may be found not in new product offerings but in a shift of the company's purpose to a higher plane. Precisely defining a company's purpose can also be a competition differentiator. It helps clarify your company in the marketplace.

Identifying our personal purpose is often more difficult than figuring out one for a business. We can be confronted with redefining our purpose when we face a life transition.

A lost relationship, a lost job or simply passing a milestone birthday can disrupt our personal sense of purpose.

Optimizing our personal purpose also takes time. It can take months, years or even decades. Don't give up. Keep searching. Living our most vital life requires us to have a framework and some tools to construct or reconstruct our purpose during these transition times. That is where the concept of dreaming greatly comes into play which we discuss in the next lesson.

DREAM GREATLY

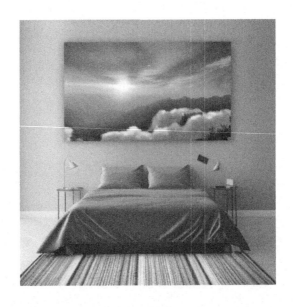

"Go Confidently in the Direction of Your Dreams"

Henry David Thoreau

Take a fierce first step.

Make time to contemplate your purpose. Too often we run through life and never think about our present purpose or what we would like it to be. Don't be that person. Set aside 1000 seconds today (about 17 minutes) and pursue clarity about your purpose for being on the planet.

Begin by silencing the voice of judgment in your head.

I have cared for hundreds of elite athletes and C-suite executives during my surgical career. They are no different than the rest of us. They all face serious personal or family issues. They all have challenges. They are all vulnerable in some way. What they have in common is an ability to silence the voice of judgment in their head. They can will themselves into believing they can achieve anything. They also have developed a staggering capacity to metabolize pain and uncertainty. They are like alchemists. They can turn pain and uncertainty into power. They use pain to fuel the missions that help fulfill their purpose. Let's listen to how one person ignites his vitality.

"I smell greatness." That's how NFL Hall of Famer Ronnie Lott started his remarks. He looked directly into the 250 eyes in the audience and said it again: "I smell greatness." He was speaking to a group of former elite collegiate football players. He knew what it was like to feel doubtful about his abilities. When he started his collegiate career at the University of Southern California (USC), he was overwhelmed. He thought he didn't belong with his highly recruited teammates. He knew he had to rise to another level in order to survive. The young former football players in the audience were stellar collegiate athletes, but they were not good enough to play professionally. They had to find a life after football. Lott reminded them we are constantly transitioning. We face new concerns daily. We are insecure about our future. We may not feel prepared for the next week, day, or minute.

Lott then challenged the assembled group. He shared his personal mantra: "Let's Go." He repeats that simple sentence to himself over and over again. He started saying that to himself on his first day at USC football practice. He quietly said to himself, "Let's Go" as he lined up to cover a speedy wide receiver. He was reminding himself he could do it. He was silencing the voice of judgment in his head that he would fail or he did not belong on the team. He continues to use that simple phrase every day to motivate himself. He also reminds us to simply get moving toward our goals.

Let's go face each day with strength. Let's go fight our fears. Let's go help others. Let's go be great. Lott's professional purpose now is to inspire people to believe in themselves. He knows inertia is one of the biggest barriers to greatness. People simply fail to get started. We can be the reason we fail. We can list many reasons why we may fail. We unfortunately discount the many reasons why we may succeed. This leads to paralysis. Many people would rather not try than try and fail.

So, get out of your own way and follow Lott's simple mantra. Say to yourself, "Let's Go." Get moving toward identifying your purpose. Set a specific set of goals. Make progress toward those goals every day. Once you overcome the iner-tia, momentum will carry you forward.

Dream Greatly

Pause for a moment and tame the wilderness in your mind. Think only about what you would do if you optimally spent your time and energy. That is your peak purpose. Set an inten-tion to define it. Stretch out toward that purpose. Close your eyes for a minute and contemplate that purpose. Write down your thoughts and ideas. Don't judge them. Dream greatly as you search for your peak purpose. Dreaming greatly helps you define your purpose by focusing your effort. It helps you eliminate many of the activities and actions in your life that are distracting you from your purpose. It tidies up your life.

Dreaming greatly also expresses faith in your own abilities. Why not bet on yourself? The minute you bet on yourself, your confidence soars. Believing in yourself is contagious. It also helps other people believe in you.

Don't seek to live other people's dreams. Develop and live your own dreams. You may be ridiculed for being audacious. Ignore the critics. Set your gaze to the galaxies. Do so with a willingness to endure some suffering. No one reaches the mountaintop without developing some blisters. Realize working toward a difficult goal also has intrinsic value. You will know later in life you did your best with your time on Earth. Remember, you may inspire other people with your willingness to tackle difficult problems.

Listen sometime to Steve Jobs' 2005 commencement speech at Stanford. He had many specific sage suggestions about how to pursue one's purpose. Here are three:

- "Your time is limited, so don't waste it living someone else's life."
- "Have the courage to follow your heart and intuition."
- "Stay hungry, stay foolish."

Defining your peak purpose is a daunting task. It means taking responsibility for your actions. It demands brutal honesty. The process may take days, months, or even years. Stop gorging yourself on excuses. Abandon victimhood. Set sail toward a distant shining shore. Sometimes it requires a jolt, a shock, or even devastation to awaken you to your peak purpose. Eliminating what you don't want to be helps you become what you want to be. Pursuing your peak purpose produces the most total vitality in your life. Failing to execute on your peak purpose results in a vitality gap.

This gap is the amount of vitality you could be experiencing if you lived for your peak purpose instead of your present purpose. The chart below helps explain this concept.

The Vitality Gap

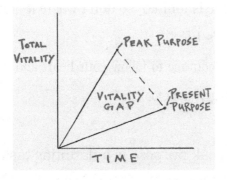

The longer you spend trying to fulfill your peak purpose, the more overall vitality you will experience. A peak purpose is also precise. It doesn't try to accomplish everything. It tries to execute on what you uniquely can achieve. Your peak purpose should consist of a short sentence, no more than eight words.

Channel Your Inner Hemingway

"For sale: Baby shoes, never worn." This six-word flash fiction story is often attributed to Ernest Hemingway. That may or may not be true. Hemingway's philosophy was to be concise but also convey a profound message.

Seek to do the same with your peak purpose statement. Being economical with your purpose statement forces you to focus. It helps you say no to anything that does not help you push your purpose forward.

A final way to dream greatly and identify your peak purpose is to participate in your passions. This means to play. It means to spend some of your precious time just having fun doing the things you love to do. Playing and having fun remind us we can do anything with our lives. They resurrect our inner child who was an expert in dreaming greatly.

I bleed maize and blue because I hold two degrees from the University of Michigan. ("Maize and blue" are the school's famous colors.) I embraced the university with unparalleled enthusiasm during my many years on campus. I was blessed to obtain a stellar education and also had a fantastic time.

Now, I love watching Michigan football and basketball games. I am not just a fan. I am a zealot when it comes to anything Michigan. I never realized this passion would provide me with a great opportunity to spread my message of vitality.

A couple years ago, I traveled back to Ann Arbor and was invited by the Michigan basketball coaches to talk about my vitality work after practice. I remembered Ronnie Lott's awesome speech and did my best to inspire the elite athletes. Below is a small portion of what I said to them.

Great people are excellent managers of their time. They take calculated chances with their time. Great people also play the game of life thinking of time like poker chips. They commit their time chips only to worthy causes. Great people commit their time to tackling difficult, sometimes impossible, tasks. They search for opportunities to demonstrate calm in the middle of a storm. Great people are also slow to get angry. They don't waste their precious time complaining or gossiping. Great people value relationships over almost anything else. And, they have a bias toward action.

I believe we all have greatness within us. We all have the ability to dream greatly. The question for all of us is: What will we choose to do with that greatness?

Still struggling with your purpose? Then consider following these seven steps that incorporate much of the last two lessons.

Step One: Reflect on your Values and Passions

- Think about what you are passionate about.
- What causes or issues do you care about?
- What activities give you a sense of fulfillment or joy?

Step Two: Explore Your Strengths and Skills

- Think about what you are naturally good at or what you have trained yourself to do well.
- What are your top talents and abilities?
- How can you use them to make a positive impact on the world?

Step Three: Get Out of Your Comfort Zone

- Take on new challenges and try new things.
- You may discover a new passion or talent that you never knew you had.

Step Four: Seek Guidance and Mentorship

- Talk to people you respect and admire, and ask them about their own journey to find their purpose.
- Learn from their experiences and wisdom.

Step Five: Experiment, Review and Revise

- Do not be afraid to try different things or test different hypotheses. It's okay if you make mistakes and have to start over.
- You may not find your purpose immediately. It may take some time and experimentation to discover what truly resonates with you.
- Expect you will need to review and revise your purpose over time.

Step Six: **Think How to Serve Others with Your Purpose**

- Think about how your purpose can serve not only your own happiness but also that of the people around you, and society as a whole.
- Seek to Serve

Step Seven: Reflect and Keep Track of Your Progress

- Keep track of your thoughts and experiences in a journal, it can help you reflect on your journey and progress.

It's important to remember is that your purpose may evolve over time, and it's okay if you don't have all the answers right away.

The important thing is to stay open-minded and continue the process of a lifelong exploration of why you are here on the planet.

Exercise 7

In eight words or less, try to articulate your purpose statements.

(They can be merged into one single statement.)

1. Personal Purpose:

2. Professional Purpose:

Don't forget to nourish yourself as you pursue your peak purpose. Start a list of how you could nourish your physical, mental, social, and spiritual well-being. Try to identify two ways to nourish yourself for each of the four pillars. Below are some examples to consider. There are, however, literally thousands of possible options. We will discuss many of these in greater detail later in the book.

Vitality Nourishment Options

Physical

- Prioritize sleep
- Stretch your hamstrings daily
- Go for a walk twice a week
- Ride an exercise bike three times per week
- Take a yoga, dance, strength or spin class
- Lose five pounds over the next two months

Mental

- Turn your phone off for one hour per day
- Write down five things you are grateful for today
- Schedule a 10-minute tranquility timeout every day
- Practice deep breathing exercises
- Listen to a great book while you commute
- Avoid assholes whenever possible
- Put inspirational quotes on your bathroom mirror
- Take a one-day screen vacation

Social

- Listen intently when your spouse or partner is speaking
- Call an old friend and catch up
- Reach out and spend time with a group that may be socially isolated
- Organize a dinner with friends
- Hang out with people who you want to be friends with
- Plan a trip with some friends from school
- Reconnect with a family member
- Go to a concert or comedy club with friends

Spiritual

- Serve someone in need this week
- Take a long walk or hike alone without your phone
- Send a care package with a thankful message to a friend
- Identify a cause you want to contribute to with your time, talent, or treasure
- Go to a religious service

Spiritual

- Meditate or pray daily
- Fast for 12 hours
- Forgive someone who has wronged you
- Write a letter to your future self to be opened on your next birthday

Exercise 8

Write down two specific ways to nourish yourself per category.

Physical

1.

2.

Mental

1.

2.

Social

1.

2.

Spiritual

1.

2.

CONSIDER SLEEP A SUPERPOWER

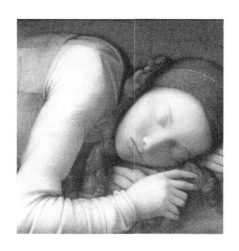

"A Well-Spent Day Brings Happy Sleep."

Leonardo Da Vinci

W hat do Tom Brady, Serena Williams, and Roger Federer have in common? They are all elite, age-defying athletes. They also gorge themselves on a legal performance-enhancing drug called sleep when they were competing. We should follow their example. Society is starting to celebrate sleep instead of praising people who brag about how little they sleep. The reason is simple. Sleep is a superpower. It helps athletes perform better. Optimal sleep is also associated with a longer life, better academic performance, and better-looking skin. The collective conversation has shifted from why we should sleep to how can we enhance our sleep.

Sleep is crucial to our vitality but many questions remain such as:

- Why do we sleep for up to a third of our lives?
- Where did the eight hours of sleep rule come from?
- What is the history of sleep?

The precise reason why we sleep has yet to be fully understood. We do know, however, that sleep is more important than food and that all animals must sleep to survive. This makes sleep the foundation of our physical and mental well-being. Poor sleep also impairs our immune system, our cardiovascular system and most importantly our brains.

Let's begin by defining sleep. It is a state of consciousness associated with limited interactions with our surroundings. This is a very odd thing to do in general. That's why I'm still baffled as to why we sleep.

Researchers have tried to explain why sleep is mandatory. Here are a few theories:

- Sleep is required to restore function. It allows for the body to relax and repair itself.
- The brain plasticity theory suggests sleep is required to help wire the brain and that sleep helps us learn. Newly published data also suggests sleep helps the brain flush out waste products. This means sleep may really help you clear you head.

- The energy conservation theory follows the data that we burn less calories when we sleep. This decreases the need to find and consume food.

My take on sleep is we need a fundamental breakthrough to truly understand its pivotal role to living a vital life.

Not all sleep is the same. There are many stages of sleep. Researchers study how long people are in each stage. No one to my knowledge has identified the precise number of hours that is optimal or how much time is spent in each stage. It varies by person. It is partially related to your genes and the mechanisms that control your internal or circadian clock.

An interesting historical finding is the concept of two sleep times. Prior to the revolution of electric lighting, most people slept for about four hours. They then engaged in some activity for about an hour and then slept for another four hours. Published historical records found over 500 references to "segmented sleep." The idea of eight straight hours of sleep as the ideal for everyone is hotly debated. Sleep also varies with age. Babies sleep extensively. Older people dream of sleeping like babies.

We know one thing for sure: poor sleep is terrible for your mind and body. Even a single day of not sleeping well can impact your vitality. Some researchers believe we can pay back a sleep debt. Other researchers are skeptical about sleeping on the weekends to make up for poor sleep during the week.

Too often we ignore sleep. We minimize its value. Don't be that person. Commit to putting sleep near the top of your To Do list instead of hoping to fit it into your life. Decide what you may have to cut out of your day in order to sleep better. Remember what we learned in Lesson One about thinking with time in mind.

Identify at least one thing you can stop doing to make more time to sleep. This could be reducing social media time or cutting out a streaming video show. It could be whining or gossiping. Find 15 or 30 minutes in your day that you are wasting. Everyone has a life leak that is sapping his or her vitality.

Use that time to optimize your sleep. This is an example of proactively designing your day and part of an effective sleep action plan.

A sleep action plan can be broken down into two components: relaxation strategies and sleep hygiene. Relaxation is crucial to sleep. Relaxation means to be free of tension and anxiety. This is a difficult state to achieve in our world today and it is killing our sleep. What interferes with the total amount and quality of our sleep isn't always obvious. That's where a sleep diary can help you. Begin your diary by recording some simple parameters. An example of a simple sleep diary is outlined below:

Sleep Diary with Two Examples

- Lights Out Time:
- Wake Up Time:
- Total "Sleep" Time:
- Sleep Quality:
- Comments:

Monday

- Lights Out Time: 11 pm
- Wake Up Time: 7 am
- Total "Sleep" Time: 8 hours
- Sleep Quality: 8 / 10
- Comments: Exercised at lunch

Tuesday

- Lights Out Time: 11:30 pm
- Wake Up Time: 6 am
- Total "Sleep" Time: 6.5 hours
- Sleep Quality: 4 / 10
- Comments: Too much work stress

Patterns will begin to emerge if you keep track for a week. This will help optimize your sleep. An example of a sleep diary in a spreadsheet format is seen in the figure below.

Exercise 9

Complete a sleep diary for a full week.

Day	Lights Out	Wake Up	Total Time	Quality (0 -10)	Comments
Sun					
Mon					
Tues					
Wed					
Thur					
Fri					
Sat					

You may find your work is the primary stress generator that interferes with your sleep. Or, you may find specific actions such as exercise mitigate your stress and help you sleep better. Music or meditation are other ways to reduce stress and relax. Consider finding ways to relax and quiet your mind as a critical assignment. It is a crucial component of a sleep action plan. Here are my top five relaxation strategies:

Top Five Relaxation Strategies

1. Exercise consistently (Walk, run, go to the gym, just MOVE)
2. Write down your "Things To Do" before going to bed
3. Listen to calming music
4. Meditation, breathing exercises, and/or prayer
5. Go outside and enjoy nature

Exercise is at the top of the list because it may be the best way to enhance sleep. It burns off excess energy. For me it is a reset button. I go to the gym if I cannot let something go that is bothering me about work. Pushing myself at the gym forces the work-related issues out of my immediate consciousness. I can only focus on how fast I am running or how hard I am pedaling on a spin bike. Exercising hard quiets my mind.

Writing down what you need to do for the next day on a piece of paper is my second relaxation suggestion. I have been doing this for years without any supporting evidence.

It was just a habit I had developed. Then I found a study supporting the idea. Dr. Michael Scullin, director of Baylor University's Sleep Neuroscience and Cognition Laboratory, conducted a controlled trial. He and his colleagues found that people who wrote down a list of things to do fell asleep faster and slept better than people who wrote down a list of completed tasks. His data supports the hypothesis that writing down things to do offloads anxious thoughts and reduces worry.

Music can also be a powerful way to relax you. Many of us have playlists to amp us up when we exercise. I suggest creating a calm playlist. Pick songs you know help soothe your mind, body, and soul. This can be any type of music that helps relax you. Dozens of mobile applications have also been scientifically developed to help you sleep using a variety of music and sounds. Just think of music as another tool that you can use to enhance your sleep.

Meditating, breathing exercises, and/or praying before bed can also help calm your mind and prepare you for sleep. I do a combination of all three almost every day. I also use deep breathing exercises to help me go back to sleep if I wake up in the middle of the night. At first, I was skeptical. Now, I am convinced. Try doing three sets of 10 deep breaths in and out and see if helps you. The cost is zero and the payoff may be better sleep.

The fifth suggestion to help you relax is to get outside. Many of us spend less time outside and more time inside cocooned in a 68-to-72 degree-controlled environment. Go outside, especially if it is hot or cold. Dress appropriately, but let your body experience some temperature and humidity. Walk on some grass in your bare feet. Go for a walk in a park with trees. Simply being outside in nature helps to calm us despite the challenges of temperature change.

Sleep hygiene is the other fundamental component of a sleep action plan. These are common sense recommendations that we often ignore. Review the list below and seek to optimize each parameter. Add in your own ways to improve your sleep hygiene.

Eight Sleep Hygiene Recommendations

1. Set a consistent sleep/wake schedule
2. Optimize your sleep environment. Make it cool, dark, and quiet. (E.g., fan, dark shades, sleep mask, ear plugs)
3. Banish your phone from your bedroom
4. Limit exposure to screens after 8 pm
5. Limit intake of caffeine and alcohol
6. No eating or drinking two hours before bed
7. Get an awesome pillow that you love
8. Try aromatherapy to relax you into sleep

Ignore the sirens of stupidity calling you to sleep less. Seek to identify your ideal amount of sleep. Then, make sleep sacrosanct.

Exercise 10

Complete your Sleep Action Plan

Record Your Top Two Relaxation Strategies

1.

2.

Record Your Top Two Sleep Hygiene Things to Execute

1.

2

LESSON SIX

STOCKPILE HEALTH

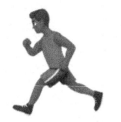 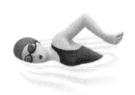 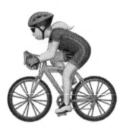

*"Some people WANT it to happen, some WISH it
would happen, others MAKE it happen."*
Michael Jordan

Stockpiling physical health focuses on engaging in consistent exercise over long periods of time. It helps us minimize (or even avoid) some of the decline in function associated with aging. Too often we wait until we experience an injury to start a physical therapy-type routine. Or, we go to the gym because our doctors told us to. This may be after finding out we had elevated blood pressure or high cholesterol.

It is much better to be proactive and seek out ways to stockpile physical health. It can help you avoid injuries. Long-term data supports the concept. In one study, people in their 70s who had exercised for decades had muscle tissue that was indistinguishable under a microscope from 30-year-old muscle tissue. This data proves it is a myth that all our systems decline with age. Not everything is under our control but we will live much more vital lives if we choose to stockpile physical health by consistently exercising.

We are also bombarded with advertising about the importance of saving enough money for retirement. We are encouraged to put away as much money as we can for our "golden years." We have been told about the value of compounded interest for our financial health. Put away $5000 as an initial investment and contribute $100 a month to a retirement plan at 5% interest compounded annually; 20 years later you will have over $50,000 saved. Financial stability is important but so is your health. What most people ignore is that your "golden years" will be miserable if you do not have your health.

Imagine speaking to yourself five, 10, or 40 years from now. What would you say? I recommend respecting your future self. One critical way you can do this is to begin to stockpile physical health. Too often we focus on stockpiling wealth. But wealth can't buy health.

Consider making regular contributions to a *Vitality Bank Account (VBA)*. Meaningful physical contributions to your *VBA* are specific actions that improve your flexibility, strength, and endurance (including deep breathing). These contributions pay dividends as you age. Calculating how much health you will compound by consistently exercising is not as easy as financial planning, but the same concept applies. The sooner you start stockpiling physical health, the more benefits you will reap. So, start today. Start stockpiling health. Your future self will thank you.

Let's explore some specific ways to stockpile physical health. Start by simply moving every day. Make it a priority. Don't let exercise become an afterthought. Once you have set an intention to exercise, make a specific plan.

Mondays may be a killer day at work or school for you. Plan ahead and make time for 15 minutes of stretching or a short walk in the middle of that day instead of eliminating exercise completely.

Focus on setting up your schedule to exercise vigorously at least three days a week. I can hear the excuse machine cranking up: "I don't have time to exercise." "I'm too busy." "I have three kids to take care of." "I'm too old to exercise." "I don't know what to do." The list could go on forever. Ignore those demons in your head. Transform those excuses into barriers and then overcome those barriers with determination and toughness. Get creative. Take your kids on a walk or jog while pushing them in a stroller. We are never too old to exercise. The excuse about not knowing how to exercise no longer applies. There are millions of free videos online to work out almost any part of your body.

Take it to another level if you are already reasonably fit. Exercise relentlessly. Focus on flexibility first. Think of stretching like brushing your teeth. Your tendons and muscles are healthier with consistent stretching. As we get older our tendons especially become stiffer. This is a significant contributor to joint pain. Too often we emphasize strength and endurance and forget flexibility.

Your frame fitness is predictive of your overall well-being. Frame fitness includes all of your joints including your spine. These joints are supported by ligaments, tendons, cartilage and muscle.

I've been practicing orthopedic surgery now for more than 25 years in the same location. That has allowed me to witness how my patients function over a long period of time. Many have been relentless exercisers. These people are now reaping the benefits. They may be in their 60s, 70s or 80s and are still skiing, playing tennis or hiking long distances. Others have neglected their physical well-being and are now paying the price. They are having difficulty just executing on their activities of daily living. They have trouble climbing stairs or even getting out of a chair.

The good news is your musculoskeletal system is modifiable until the day you die. You can improve your strength, endurance and flexibility. It just takes effort and consistency.

Emerging research also points to the value of maintaining our frames. This is especially true about the muscles that support our spines and joints. We lose about five percent of our muscle mass per decade after the age of 30. This loss accelerates rapidly after age 60. It is not well known but decreasing grip strength is associated with an increased risk of dying.

It is therefore crucial to begin as soon as possible to maintain your muscle. The best way to improve your muscle function is to perform resistance-type exercises such as lifting weights or using devices such as a leg press machine. An exercise bike also qualifies as a resistance machine.

Aerobic training in the form of walking, hiking or running is important especially for our cardiovascular system. Recent data suggest, however, that resistance training may be even more important. This type of training can help improve the structure and quality of your bone.

Resistance training is also valuable because our muscles release proteins and molecules called myokines in response to us contracting them. Myokines have powerful effects within and beyond our muscles. This area of research is rapidly evolving but there is significant scientific support confirming resistance training helps improve our mobility, helps maintain our cognitive function, and improves glucose tolerance. All of these are vitality enhancers. One critical study found high intensity exercise reduced the incidence of highly metastatic cancers by 73% compared with being inactive. This is a staggering piece of scientific evidence that demands our attention.

Don't forget we can work on the muscles that control our breathing such as the diaphragm. These muscles can be trained by doing deep breathing exercises. You can think of deep breathing like weightlifting for your lungs.

The Bottom Line is: Muscle Matters.

Let me illustrate that point by finishing this lesson with a story. A woman in her late 70s came into my office complaining of knee pain. She was upset because she was having difficulty doing almost any type of physical activity including getting off the commode. She was particularly distressed because her husband was in excellent shape. He had been a lifelong exerciser. She hated any type of exercise.

She looked despondent when I first evaluated her. Her exam showed evidence of significant lower extremity weakness. Her balance was also terrible. Fortunately, she didn't have any knee swelling and her X-rays only showed moderate arthritis. It was clear her main problem was low muscle mass and poor muscle control.

I explained to her she had a chance to improve but it would take time and significant effort. She didn't like hearing that. She wanted a cortisone shot or something simple. I outlined a program that included quadriceps activation exercises and an exercise called: Sit-to-Stand.

In this exercise a person rises multiple times from a seated position to a standing position. This is best done with a chair that has arms in case the person needs to help propel themselves from a seated to a standing position with their arms.

My patient could barely do one repetition on her first visit with me. I asked her to try to do one or two repetitions three times per day for the next month along with the quadriceps activation exercises. She pouted about not getting a shot and reluctantly agreed to my recommendations.

She returned about six weeks later. She was not happy with me when I examined her. I, however, was excited. I could see her quadriceps tone had improved. She could now do a set of five Sit-to-Stand exercises. She still had to use her arms to help but this was meaningful progress.

I asked her to continue with the program and check back with me in a month. She looked at me with sad eyes and said she would never be able to get better. That's when I asked her to be like *The Little Engine That Could.*

I told her that book was my favorite when I was growing up. I retold the story of the small blue engine that repeated the mantra of: I think I can, I think I can. I think I can. Eventually, the little blue engine pulled a heavy load up and over a tall mountain.

I'm not sure she believed me, but she seemed to be inspired by my retelling of the story. She agreed to push forward and be consistent with her exercises.

I didn't see her for two months. She came in as my last patient of the day on a busy Monday. I dreaded going in to see her. I expected her to complain again about not being able to keep up with her fit husband and beg me for a cortisone shot. I knocked and slowly opened the door. She put up hand and told me to stop.

She then bolted out of the chair without using her arms with a beaming smile on her face. She told me that she just turned 80 and felt great. She easily did a set of 10 Sit-to-Stand exercises. She had also resumed going on walks with her husband. She was delighted and so was I.

Then, she handed me a beautiful copy of *The Little Engine That Could*. I carefully opened the front cover and saw it was a first edition, published in 1930. It wasn't a gift. She wanted to show me how much she also loved the book and its message.

She didn't say it at her previous visit, but she said thinking about the little blue engine had helped her be consistent. I asked her if I could take a picture with her and the book. That picture with both of us beaming still hangs in an exam room in my office. She has given me permission to tell anyone her story. The hope is it will inspire others to believe in themselves and the power of exercising relentlessly at any age.

Exercise 11

Commit to focusing on your physical fitness in the four categories below. List at least one way you will specifically work on each category.

1. **Flexibility**

Example: Stretch your hamstrings

2. **Strength**

Example: Use a soup can or dumbbell and do bicep curls

3. **Endurance**

Example: Walk, hike, or run three times per week

4. **Breathing**

Example: Take 10 deep breaths three times per day

STAPLE YOUR
MOUTH SHUT

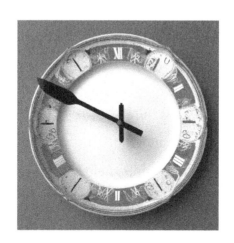

"I Fast for Greater Physical and Mental

Efficiency"

Plato

D o you want to be treated well or optimally?

Almost all doctors treat you well. The only way they can treat you optimally is for you to take ownership of your health. Seeking to live at your ideal weight is one of the most important ways to begin this process.

No one is force-feeding you. You are in charge of your food and drink choices. These choices affect not just your weight but also your risk for a variety of diseases and disorders. They also influence your mood and affect your social interactions.

Your time management skills, your level of discipline, your sense of purpose, your sleep patterns, and your willingness to engage in exercise all affect your ability to live at your ideal weight. It may seem counterintuitive, but I recommend mastering those vitality skills before tackling your weight.

Living as close as possible to your ideal weight is pivotal to vitality. Most people weigh too much. Seventy percent of people in the United States are either overweight or obese. This is a staggeringly complex problem. No one can force people to lose weight. I can cajole or perhaps inspire my family, friends, and patients to work toward their ideal weight. Each person, however, must make his or her own decisions.

This lesson will review some data about why our weight is associated with our vitality. This is for information purposes only. Please check with your personal physician before initiating any specific weight management plan.

Let me begin by dispelling with some data the excuse about arthritic knee pain as being the cause of people not being able to lose weight. I've heard it too many times to count. I can't lose weight because my knees hurt. I need a knee replacement and then I will be able to lose some weight. Here are the facts: overweight people who have their knees replaced don't lose weight. They *gain* weight. Published peer reviewed articles have shown obese patients who undergo knee replacement surgery report decreased pain scores and improvement in their function. Despite this functional improvement, they are heavier two years after the surgery.

The authors of one study concluded surgery alone is not a sufficient intervention for obesity.

Losing weight can significantly improve your knee function. Biomechanical studies have found a one-pound reduction in body weight results in a four-fold reduction in force on the knee joint. That means if you lost five pounds your knee would feel as if you lost 20 pounds. Here are some real-world testimonials about weight loss and knee pain from my students and patients. They have given me permission to share these quotes.

- "I've lost 25 pounds. Now, I can't remember when my knee hurt."
- "Losing weight made my knees feel better for sure."
- "It is amazing what you have control over as a patient."

The person who lost 25 pounds now has a knee that is transmitting 100 pounds less force through its cartilage with every step. That's why living at or near your ideal weight is so important for the treatment of knee osteoarthritis. This is also true of many other diseases such as diabetes, heart disease and cancer.

Obesity has been called a chronic relapsing condition by a variety of clinicians and researchers. Its incidence has tripled over the last 40 years to approximately two billion cases worldwide according to the World Health Organization. This organization calls obesity preventable. I agree and believe it is impossible to enhance global vitality without addressing this massive problem.

In her book, "Radical Candor," author Kim Scott argues that brutal honesty is required to help people at their work. I think her concept also applies to addressing the problem of obesity.

Start today to take responsibility for your weight. Know what you choose to eat and drink is one of the cornerstones of your vitality. Understand you can control your diet and weight at least to some degree. Search for ways to help yourself.

Let's start by identifying an intrinsic motivation. This is a difficult and personal task. Only you can answer for you. Start by finding a sustainable source of motivation. Looking better, reducing your risk of dying, and feeling better are all possible reasons to live at your ideal weight. There are many other reasons. The important thing to execute on is to identify the "why" of your weight.

You must identify your "why" if you want to treat yourself optimally. Managing your diet and weight is a skill you can master. You may be able to do so on your own. More often, you will need someone to help you. This could be a friend, family member, weight loss program or your physician.

Jettison excuses. Reframe any eating issues you may have into specific barriers. Then seek ways to overcome the barriers. Brainstorm solutions instead of complaining about how "impossible" it is to lose weight. Find a person or a group to help you be accountable for your goals. Eating a proper diet and seeking to live life at your ideal weight is a very difficult skill to master. It is also a moving target.

Losing weight is more difficult as we age because our metabolism slows down. Start measuring how many calories you truly consume every day instead of repeating excuses like, "I eat like a bird and still gain weight." Be brutally honest about the process. Weigh yourself every day at the same time and figure out precisely how many calories you need to eat to stay at an even weight. You will need to be under that number in order to lose weight. The simple act of having to step on the bathroom scale in the morning and stare at the number may be enough for some people to improve their eating habits.

So, what is one of the best ways to return to your ideal weight or at least make progress toward that goal? Here is my simple and snarky solution: Staple your mouth shut. Use that mantra to simply reduce the amount you eat if your goal is to lose weight. We cannot "out exercise" our mouths. We must work on the other side of the equation and reduce our caloric intake if we truly wish to live at our ideal weight.

The global weight management market is approaching $500 billion dollars. This money is spent on an astonishing number of diet programs, medications and surgeries. Newer medications use powerful molecules that help patients feel fuller. This leads to lower caloric intake and therefore weight loss. Surgical options include bypassing or banding the stomach. A simpler solution is to eat less and eat less often.

Time restricted eating, also known as intermittent fasting, is another approach to weight loss that is gaining popularity. There are many forms of this approach. Restricting food intake to eight hours per day is one example. This can be done by stopping any food intake at 8 pm and then not eating until noon the next day. That represents a 16 hour fast. It is then followed by an eight-hour eating window. What represents a fast is hotly debated. Some fasting programs recommend only water, others allow for flavored soda water, tea, or coffee. The data supporting intermittent fasting is rapidly evolving. It appears to be as good or better than simply restricting total calories as an approach to weight loss.

Intermittent fasting also improves outcomes for diabetes, cardiovascular disease, neurologic disorders, and even cancer.

It also suppresses inflammation and can improve circadian rhythms and sleep. There are also a slew of studies claiming fasting helps animals live longer. Human studies are ongoing. The bottom line is fasting seems to be a very good thing for your body. And it is a cost-free way of enhancing your vitality.

Unfortunately, there is much we still need to understand about how to live at our ideal weight. Here is an interesting piece of scientific data about milkshakes that illustrates this point. We first will have to learn a little physiology to understand this important work.

Ghrelin is a hormone produced by your body to signal to your brain you need to eat. When your stomach is empty, you produce more ghrelin and your appetite rises. When your stomach is full, ghrelin drops and your appetite decreases.

Now, let's dive into a study published in the *Journal of Health Psychology*. The effect of mindset on whether a person felt full after consuming two supposedly different milkshakes was investigated. The first one was labeled as "indulgent" containing 640 calories. The second was labeled "sensible" containing 140 calories. Blood samples were drawn before and after consumption of the shakes and ghrelin levels were measured. In reality, both shakes were exactly the same containing 380 calories.

Participants who thought they were consuming an "indulgent" milkshake had a steep decline in their ghrelin levels. The ones who thought they were consuming a "sensible" milkshake had a relatively flat decline in their ghrelin levels.

The study concluded ghrelin levels after food consumption are connected to a person's mindset. When we believe we are consuming something indulgent we react by lowering our ghrelin levels more than when we believe we are eating something sensible. Other research has shown that our powerful hunger hormones are affected simply by viewing pictures of food. Importantly, the level of hormone responses to visualizing food is highly variable.

Why are your ghrelin levels so important? They are crucial because elevated levels can lead to increased body weight and fat. This occurs because high ghrelin levels drive food consumption. Next time I eat broccoli I am going to label it as "indulgent" in my mind and hope my ghrelin levels plummet. Importantly, ghrelin levels rise with shorter sleep durations. This is an example of how our vitality is interconnected to a variety of parameters.

Living at your ideal weight is complicated. Future research will hopefully tell us how best to navigate this crucial component of our vitality.

Exercise 12

Identify the "why" of your weight.

Write down the top reason you want to live at your ideal weight:

Possible Answers

- "I want to look better."
- "I want to live longer."
- "I want to control my diabetes, heart disease or hypertension."
- "I want to feel better on a daily basis."

Exercise 13

Commit to living at your ideal weight.

Copy this sentence in your own handwriting on a piece of paper:

"I commit to living at my ideal weight."

Now, post that piece of paper on your bathroom mirror. Weigh yourself every day and figure out how many absolute calories you can ingest and stay at the same weight. Know that you will have to eat less than that number if you want to lose weight.

CULTIVATE CLOSENESS

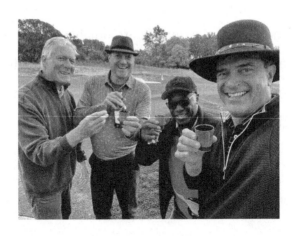

"A True Friend Accepts Who You Are,

But Also Helps You Become Who You Should Be."

Unknown

C loseness counts.
Being connected to other people is a fundamental component of our vitality. Too often we fail to recognize the importance of our social connections. The scientific data supporting closeness as a crucial vitality parameter is overwhelming.

A Harvard study of adult development is one example. This study began in 1938 by evaluating sophomores in college and tracked them over a long period of time. Interestingly, future President John F. Kennedy was one of the students in the first cohort of subjects. It is the longest running investigation of what contributes to our health and well-being spanning more than 80 years. The crucial and surprising finding was how important our social relationships are to our vitality.

The study found that close relationships were more important than money in predicting a long and happy life. Another fascinating finding was our satisfaction with our relationships at age 50 predicted our health at age 80. Loneliness was also found to be similar to smoking or alcoholism in terms

of predicting negative long-term outcomes. Other researchers have confirmed these findings. They found social inte-
gration and close relationships were more important than
physical activity, smoking or body composition. Recent
research has further associated loneliness with higher levels of inflammatory markers in our bodies. This is important because inflammation is associated to serious problems
such diabetes, heart disease and cancer. I was astonished to
learn that 40-80% of our health and wellness are connected
directly or indirectly to social factors.

The research all points in the same direction: Closeness
Counts.

Vital people recognize the importance of their connections with their friends, family, co-workers and community.
They prioritize closeness. They embrace and enjoy being
connected.

We don't have to be taught to do this when we are young.
We seek out friendships at school. We want to be part of a

group outside of our nuclear families. Later, however, we discount the value of our social fitness. We pursue money, fame, power, or other transitory tonics that fail to quench our thirst. We let our relationships wither. We fail to fertilize them when they need attention. Only as time passes do we realize our relationships are what makes life so special and precious.

So, what are we to do if we want to optimize our vitality? We reject the worldly pursuits and embrace closeness. We seek to learn how to cultivate closeness. How can we do that?

First, recognize its value. Remember, your connections with others are more important than money, smoking, drinking or even exercise. That doesn't mean these parameters don't matter. It doesn't give you a license to party with your friends and binge drink every day of the week. It does mean we need to recognize the value of relationships to our vitality.

Second, be curious about other people's lives. Practice being open-minded, nonjudgmental, and kind. Show empathy and understanding whenever possible. Seek out opportunities to connect with people who don't look or act like you. Be a bridge builder across deep divides. The world needs more people like that.

Third, forgive to rebuild relationships. Realize we all need forgiveness. Practice compromising, showing respect, and being reliable. Build trust through honest and transparency. This suggestion is simple to state and difficult to achieve. Know that forgiveness is hard but try to do it anyway. We all need to put our egos aside and admit we have wronged others. We may also need to forgive ourselves in order to move forward and reconnect.

Fourth, practice "scary sharing." Be vulnerable and share something in your life that you are worried about. Admit you don't have it all figured out. Believe another person can and will be of help to you if you ask. One important component of scary sharing is trust. We need a way to measure if someone is going to be a gossip and spread our bad news. I have a snarky solution.

Consider telling someone you have toenail fungus. It may not be true. You can, however, assess how they react and if they spread the bad news. Your trust level with them either rises or falls depending on what happens. Telling someone you have toenail fungus is just a benign example of showing a person you trust them. You may be surprised when they use your trust of them to trust you. Be prepared when someone shares intimate serious issues with you. Listen carefully, offer advice if you can, and then put the information in a virtual lock box.

Fifth, laugh and have some fun. Find people who share your passions. Schedule time with these people and then just do something you enjoy together. Realize you will not regret having more laughter in your life. Create a list of five things you love to do. Make sure you carve out time for one every week or better yet every day. Schedule some fun with friends into your life. Never discount the value to your vitality of enjoying yourself in the company of others.

Don't wait until tomorrow. Start today to work on your social vitality. Here is a simple, almost cost-free suggestion. Text three people you haven't seen in at least a month and just say hello. Tell them you are thinking about them and hope they are doing ok. Texting them will enhance their vitality. And, your vitality will rise when they hopefully reciprocate and text you back.

"Prime-time Friends"

How many "prime-time friends" do you have? How many family members do you truly trust? These people are exceptional. You are never phony with them. You are also your authentic self. You celebrate the precious present when you are with that person. You share your sorrows and your dreams. Everyone needs trusted people to lean on during life's difficult times. We thrive in the context of their counsel and guidance. Prime-time friends and close family members fulfill two of our most important vitality needs: meaningful connections and having fun.

How do we develop such relationships? Living in the now, something we learned in Lesson One, is an excellent way to cultivate closeness. It is worth repeating because it is crucial to our vitality.

Put your phone away. Look someone in the eyes during your next conversation. Focus on what they are saying. Listen with the intent of hearing the other person. This is rare in today's society. We are all distracted. We discount the value of family and friendships. When you stop and live in the now and really listen to another person, your closeness with that person rapidly rises.

Developing closeness is a vitality skill that takes time. A recent study found it takes about 50 hours to develop an acquaintance. The same investigation found it takes about 100 hours to become a friend and at least 200 hours to become a best friend. Rarely do we devote that amount of time to developing our friendships after we have finished school.

What you talk about also matters if your goal is to cultivate closeness. You must be vulnerable. This means you are willing to share both your crazy dreams and your most difficult challenges. I knew I needed to be better at this difficult skill. I live in Silicon Valley where almost everyone is wearing an ornate mask. We supposedly have it all: brilliant weather, staggering professional opportunities, and the opportunity to explore cutting-edge technology before most people on the planet.

What's missing in Silicon Valley is a sense of social and spiritual vitality. Several years ago, I started working on enhancing my social vitality by sharing more with my close friends and family. I opened up about my personal and professional challenges. Sharing some of my crazy dreams -- like writing a book about vitality -- helped me grow closer to the most important people in my life. Surprisingly, my friends started opening up to me in ways they never had before despite knowing them for decades. They shared their aspirations. They also admitted to having financial and martial difficulties. We grew closer by sharing the most intimate and challenging parts of our lives.

We need friends and family members who can help us with different aspects of our lives. This idea led me to think about developing a *Vitality Squad*. This is a group of people I can lean on when I am in need. Each person in my squad has a different level of expertise in physical, mental, social, and spiritual wellness. My vitality rises when I seek out their help in each of these areas. I also try to be part of someone else's vitality squad by offering to help whenever I can. There is an exercise at the end of this chapter that will help you develop your own vitality squad.

I'll finish this lesson with a story about my close friend, Kevin. He swam at West Point and served as a tank commander in the Army. He was a dedicated father, husband, and successful technology executive. He also was my swim coach when I had a crazy idea of starting to do triathlons in my late 30s.

Kevin was a tall, good-looking and an elite athlete. He crushed the competition in our age group when we did races together. He never judged me for barely being able to swim 1500 meters in open water. He never looked down on my pathetic heavy and rusty bike. He took me under his broad wing and made me feel like I could do anything. He was not just my friend. He was an angel and one of the most vital people on the planet.

Unfortunately, Kevin died of amyotrophic lateral sclerosis (ALS), a nasty fatal neurodegenerative disease. This is the most ironic diagnosis I have ever witnessed. He received his diagnosis about the same time I started teaching my vitality course at Stanford. He was going to be one of my expert guest speakers about how to stay fit at any age.

He was supposed to speak in the afternoon session. When we broke for lunch, he asked me to take a short walk with him. I thought we were going to discuss his talk. Instead, he started sobbing. He simply couldn't process why he was being cut down in the prime of his life with the horrors of

ALS. He literally collapsed in my arms. I did my best to console him with lame platitudes. I didn't know what to say. Why was this happening to one of my best friends and his family? What could I do to help? I was baffled.

Kevin and his family navigated the brutal waters of ALS by going through all the stages of grief—denial, anger, depression, bargaining, and (finally) acceptance. They didn't just accept the diagnosis. They embraced it. They started organizing ice bucket challenges with the local high school water polo teams. He urged the athletes he met to think of ALS as "athletes leading and serving" instead of a terrible degenerative disease. Kevin and his amazing wife also assembled a team of people to raise money for an ALS bike ride in Napa Valley, California. Kevin spoke to the other bikers and other victims of ALS at the beginning of the race:

"I'm a strong Christian. This is a day the Lord has made. Let us rejoice and be glad. I was blessed with ALS. The blessing of having ALS is you get a community of people trying to support you. It's amazing. Imagine what we have done. We don't do it by ourselves, we do it as a community."

That day, Kevin, his wife, and their team raised over $156,000 for ALS research. He also inspired his friends and family with his faith. It is a terrible question to contemplate. What would you do if you were diagnosed with ALS? It is a question many of the people who knew him began to contemplate. Would I react in the same way? Would I embrace the diagnosis? Would I rally my friends, colleagues, and family to raise money? Or, would I retreat into a sea of despair? I'd like to think I could be like Kevin but I'm not sure how I would react.

Kevin passed at the height of the COVID pandemic in early 2021. He fought his horrific disease valiantly. I attended his funeral outside in his backyard with a small group of family and friends. It was a beautiful tribute to an amazing man that finished with the playing of Taps by an Army honor guard. The song is played on a solo bugle and is just 24 notes long. It invokes a profound sense of sadness deep in one's soul for the loss of the departed. At the end of the song, the honor guard presented Kevin's family with a perfectly folded American flag as we watched through tear-soaked eyes.

I didn't know it at the time but I would attend three more funerals of close family members and friends over the next year. The funerals were difficult but also instructive. Here are four lessons I learned from the speakers who were celebrating their departed loved ones.

- Live in the moment to make a memory last a lifetime.
- Life has to end, but love does not.
- Pursue significance not success.
- The future can dissolve in a moment.

I have always believed I won't know when my last best day would be. I need to remind myself of that every day. It helps me focus. It helps me answer these questions:

- What do I want to do with my life?
- Who do I want to spend it with?

- How do I want to be remembered?
- What can I do with my remaining time to make a difference?

The primary lesson I learned is our closeness with others is all that counts at the end of our lives. It reminds me to invest in cultivating that closeness whenever possible every day.

Exercise 14

Develop your personal "Vitality Squad."

Name one person in each of these areas who you will seek out to help you when you are in need.

Physical Vitality:

Mental Vitality:

Social Vitality:

Spiritual Vitality:

Exercise 15

Be part of someone else's "Vitality Squad."

Start by thinking about how you can best help other people. Then, reach out to at least one person with that need this week.

SERVING SPARKS HOPE

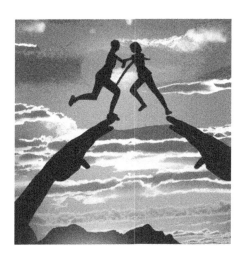

"Be a Giver Not a Taker"

Adam Grant

Reach out today with a helping hand. Reach out and serve someone in need. Reach out knowing that even in times of despair each of us has the potential to help another human.

Serving others sparks hope. It sparks hope in the person being served and it sparks hope in the server. These two components of the Vitality Octagon are closely intertwined. Serving others gives us a sense of fulfillment that fosters hope. Seeing the positive impact of our service can also improve our sense of hope. Finally, serving others and helping them overcome adversity may inspire other people to follow our example.

I have found it difficult to teach my students and clients how to have more hope. I did, however, find a correlation between a sense of purpose and having a high sense of hope. This means the higher your sense of purpose the more likely you will be to report having a high sense of hope. That correlation led me to focus on helping people identify their peak purpose. Hope should rise when we are focused on executing our highest possible purpose.

Studies have found serving others lowers blood pressure, decreases stress, and leads to higher levels of happiness. Serving and giving can also lead to what has been called the "Helper's High." Some studies have found giving can lead to a longer life even after controlling for age, exercise, and bad habits such as smoking. Interestingly, giving leads to the release of mood-related hormones such as serotonin, dopamine, and oxytocin. Giving has been associated with stimulation of the reward center in the brain known as the mesolimbic pathway. This can lead to the release of the body's natural version of morphine: endorphins. Finally, selfless volunteering has also been associated with living longer and more fulfilling lives. The hope is this scientific data will encourage all of us to serve more and take less.

Too often we forget how important it is to make time to help others. We are too caught up in our own concerns. Schedule some time to help others in need especially if you are always busy. Helping other humans is an intrinsically valuable use of your precious time. It will also help you put your own issues into perspective.

Serving others seems like a counterintuitive vitality skill. Why wouldn't I work on myself first if I want to elevate my sense of well-being? The ironic truth is focusing on someone other than yourself is a primary step toward vitality. Serving others consistently also leads to a meaningful life. And, meaning in life is a source of hope. Friedrich Nietzsche said it best: "He who has a why to live for can bear almost any how." Meaning is our why. It helps us endure whatever circumstances we face in life.

Serving and believing are closely connected spiritual vitality enhancers. We all need someone to believe in us. Sometimes, I can't find anyone to believe in me. That's when I remember God always believes in me. That is one of the reasons I believe in Him. Spirituality for me is a belief in almighty God. This is my personal choice. I am not advocating for everyone to follow my path. My faith has not always been consistent, but I have dozens of specific examples of God guiding me in times of difficulty and in times of joy. It has been my experience that I am closer to God in challenging times. Praying, going to church, and reading the Bible all boost my sense of spiritual vitality. It is also significantly enhanced by serving others whenever possible.

Spiritual vitality can be religious but does not have to be. People working to support important causes or serving others outside of religious organizations are equally enhancing their spiritual vitality. Spirituality is an adjective that means, "relating to or affecting the human spirit or soul as opposed to material or physical things." A simple definition for spirituality is a belief in something bigger than yourself. There are infinite ways to explore spirituality. The point is to value spirituality as a crucial component of your overall vitality.

Start today by believing in something bigger than yourself. Service and belief are core elements of the spiritual pillar of vitality. Without a belief in something bigger than yourself, you will miss out on what I call the *Superman* or *Wonder Woman* of vitality enhancers. It's simple: serving others dramatically enhances your own vitality. Serving others can also be your ladder out of an abyss.

Superman and Wonder Woman focus their powers on helping people in need. I believe each of us has a Superman or Wonder Woman within. We may not be able to fly like they can but we all have the ability to identify the needs of others. I also believe superheroes derive at least some of their mystical powers from helping people. So, start today and serve someone in need. You will enhance their vitality and yours.

I'll finish this lesson with the inspiring story of Hotel de Zink. I've served at this hotel for many years. It is a special emergency shelter for guests who are homeless. The hotel functions as a support structure under the guidance of church members and an organization called *Life Moves*. It is not really a hotel but rather a place that moves around each month and provides meals, shelter, and assistance. November is the month when my church serves as the "hotel."

The roots of Hotel de Zink go back to 1931 and the height of the Great Depression in the United States. Unemployment was over 25%. Many people were desperate for food and shelter. The town of Palo Alto stepped up and donated an old warehouse to serve as a shelter for people in distress. A fancy expensive hotel now sits on this prime piece of property directly across the street from the Stanford University campus.

The shelter was named the Hotel de Zink in honor of Police Chief Howard Zink, an enthusiastic supporter of helping people in need. It had a double meaning because the building was constructed of steel galvanized with zinc. During a six-month period from the fall of 1932 to the spring of 1933, the shelter housed over 9000 men, served over 40,000 meals, and gave out almost 1000 pairs of shoes. There was even a small hospital run for free by Dr. John Silliman. Palo Alto had created a place of refuge for its most needy residents. The shelter closed in 1934 after fulfilling its mission but was recently reborn as an emergency shelter that rotates among local churches.

I met an amazing guest while eating Thanksgiving dinner one year at the Hotel de Zink. Her name is Athena. She had a quick smile, bright brown eyes, and a hat that made me think of a jazz dancer. The hat was jet black and adorned with flashy sequins. We talked briefly about her cool hat. I noticed her awesome smile widen as we chatted. She then asked me pointed question.

"What's the most powerful force in the universe?"

How about that for a Thanksgiving dinner question? It staggered me a little. I paused before I answered. I wasn't sure where this conversation was going. The immediate answer in my head was love. Then, I remembered I was in a church that was presently functioning as a homeless shelter. Shouldn't the answer be God?

I decided to go with my immediate thought and said love. Athena smirked a little and then said. "Of course, it is love! And, since God IS love then He is the also the most powerful force in the universe."

I've been going to church my entire life. I've never heard a more profound and inspiring definition of God. That definition also came from a wonderful but unexpected source. That moment with Athena is seared in my memory. I came on Thanksgiving to the Hotel de Zink to serve but it was me who was served by my new friend Athena.

There are many ways to serve other people and spark hope. Here are some options to consider:

- Volunteer at a charity or non-profit organization.
- Be a mentor by sharing your knowledge and experience.
- Help friends and family simply by being available when a time of need arises.
- Perform random acts of kindness. These are small often unexpected things that improve another person's life.
- Build a sense of community by being friendly and supportive of the people around you.

There is no perfect way to help others. Just listen to your heart and be authentic.

Exercise 16

Commit today to serving others in need.

List two ways you will serve others and spark hope in the next week.

1.

2.

CONCLUSION

BECOMING A VITALITY EXPLORER

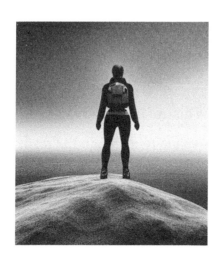

"What You Seek is Seeking You."

Rumi

Y ou may now consider yourself a *Vitality Explorer* because you have made it to the end of this book. Together we have learned many important lessons.

We have learned that time, discipline, purpose, and sleep are all essential elements that contribute to our vitality.

Time is our most precious resource that once spent cannot be regained. We have learned to live in the now, treat our seconds as precious, and write our future headlines.

Discipline is also crucial to our vitality. It helps us stay focused and execute on our top priorities. Without discipline we drift into meaningless distractions and fail to achieve our goals. We also need discipline to maintain the many habits that are essential to our vitality.

Purpose is the foundation of our vitality. It gives us meaning and direction. It helps motivate us and leads to greater satisfaction and fulfillment in life. Knowing our purpose also helps us manage our time and To Do list. We can say "No" more often and focus our effort on what we believe are the most important reasons we are on this planet.

Sleep is often ignored but a critical component of both our physical and mental well-being. Poor sleep is associated with a weaker immune system, heart disease, and depression. Vital people make sleep a top priority.

We have also learned that fitness, closeness, service, and hope are important factors that contribute to our sense of vitality.

Physical and emotional fitness are both important and connected. Engaging in regular aerobic exercise and resistance training help not only our musculoskeletal system but also our heart health, our brain health, and our mental health. It can reduce our risk of other chronic diseases and help us live longer and more productive lives. Importantly, it can help us cope with stress and reduce our anxiety.

Closeness with others is like sleep. It is too often ignored in the context of our vitality. We need to make time to build and maintain our relationships if we want to live our most vital lives. Strong relationships provide a sense of belonging and connection. These are essential for both our physical and mental well-being. Our social support systems help us cope with adversity which is an inevitable component of life. Closeness also helps us develop trust, empathy, and understanding. All of these are components of vitality.

Service, or giving back to others, is rewarding for the one that is served and also for the person providing the help. Consistently serving others improves our sense of self-worth and reinforces our purpose. It can also boost our mood and alleviate stress.

Finally, hope or maintaining a positive outlook on life is associated with a higher sense of vitality. This component of the vitality octagon is the most difficult one to teach. Hope rises when we work on all of the other vitality parameters. It is the byproduct of taking ownership over your decisions and choices. It also rises when we take action to improve our lives instead of remaining passive. Hope is also a belief that we have agency in this life. We can make a positive difference in our own lives and the lives of other people. Remember, hope is also closely connected to our sense of purpose.

It's now time to put all the lessons together into a coherent vitality action plan.

Remember how we started with the *Four Pillars of Vitality*, the *Vitality Octagon* and the *Four Zones of Living*?

Review the previous exercises embedded in this book. Are you thinking with time in mind, doubling down on discipline, pinpointing your peak purpose, dreaming greatly, considering sleep a superpower, stockpiling health, stapling your mouth shut, cultivating closeness, and sparking hope by serving? Did you complete the exercises in this book? What did you write for your future headlines? Are you nour- ishing yourself by making regular deposits into your *Vitality Bank Account* (VBA)?

It is my hope that the lessons and exercises in this book have been meaningful. Please consider sharing what- ever you may have learned with your friends, family and co-workers. Remember: the most important way to enhance your vitality is to set an intention to do so.

Set that intention knowing we all need to review and revise our vitality action plans. We need to adapt to new information that can help us lead our best life. We need to embrace the challenges we will face as we navigate the seasons of life.

We need to continue to be Vitality Explorers and engage each of our days with one simple but powerful mantra: **Dare To Be Vital.**

Exercise 17

Complete Your Personalized Vitality Action Plan.

List two specific, actionable personalized vitality recommendations for each of the four pillars.

Physical

1.

2.

Mental

1.

2.

Social

1.

2.

Spiritual

1.

2.

NOTES AND REFERENCES

Lesson One: Think with Time in Mind

Social Security has a somewhat morbid website that you can check out to see your projected number of years left to live. Check it to motivate yourself to optimize your precious seconds.
https://www.ssa.gov/oact/STATS/table4c6.html

Read more about how to Respect Your Future. This article discusses how we have better physical, mental, and financial well-being when we are more closely connected to our future selves.

Reiff, JS,Hershfield,HE, Quoidbach J. Identity over time: Perceived similarity between selves predicts well-being 10 years later. *Soc Psychol Personal Sci* 2020;11(2):160-7.

Book Suggestion: Essentialism: The Disciplined Pursuit of Less by Greg McKeown

This book helped me optimize my time. It forced me to prioritize. It helped me say no more often to what was less important and yes more often to what I valued most in life.

Quotes from the book:

"Make decisions by design not default."

"You can do anything but not everything."

Lesson Two: Double Down on Discipline

Read more about Dr. Condoleezza Rice and the privilege of struggling:
Henderson Blunt, S. 'The privilege of struggle.' How Rice understands suffering and prayer. *Christianity Today* September 1, 2003.

Kara Lawson on Handling Hard Better:
https://www.youtube.com/watch?v=oDzfZOfNki4

Book Suggestion: Discipline is Destiny by Ryan Holiday
The book discusses Stoic philosophy and how it applies to our modern life. Holiday gives his readers excellent specific examples of how to embrace discipline as a pathway to a better life.

Quotes from the book:

"In a world of distraction, focusing is a superpower."

"Discipline isn't just endurance and strength. It's also finding the best, most economical way of doing something."

Lesson Three: Pinpoint Your Peak Purpose

Check out the "Get Busy Living or Get Busy Dying" clip from The Shawshank Redemption: https://www.youtube.com/watch?v=tLpyklFEahs

Alimujiang A, Wiensch A, Boss J, et al. Association between life purpose and mortality among US adults older than 50 years. *JAMA Netw Open* 2019;2(5):e194270.

Book Suggestion: Man's Search for Meaning by Victor Frankl This is a must-read book for anyone in search of purpose. Frankl helps us realize purpose can be found in suffering. Purpose can be found in serving others. Purpose can be found when we let go of our ego. It is a profound book with many meaningful insights.

Quotes from the book:

"Suffering ceases to be suffering at the moment it finds a meaning."

"The last of one's freedoms is to choose one's attitude in any given circumstance."

Lesson Four: Dream Greatly

The "Let's Go" quote is from Ronnie Lott's speech at the Campbell Trophy Summit in 2018. For more information about the summit, follow this link: https://www.youtube.com/watch?v=3c5lAdJqvqQ

Steve Jobs' Stanford Commencement Speech: https://www.youtube.com/watch?v=UF8uR6Z6KLc

"For sale: Baby shoes, never worn" has been attributed to Ernest Hemingway. This may or may not be true. *The New Yorker* has some other interesting other six-word stories that Hemingway supposedly wrote.

Wortman, Z. Ernest Hemingway's six-word sequels. *The New Yorker* September 11, 2016.

President Teddy Roosevelt's "Man in the Arena"

McCarthy E. Roosevelt's "The Man in the Arena." *Mentalfloss.com* April 23, 2015.

Lesson Five: Consider Sleep a Superpower

Read more about why poor sleep increases the risk of dying.

Yin J, Jin X, Shan Z, et al. Relationship of sleep duration with all-cause mortality and cardiovascular events: A systematic review and dose-response meta-analysis of prospective cohort studies. *J Am Heart Assoc* 2017;6(9);e005947.

Sleep Disorders and Alzheimer's Disease.
National Institutes of Health. Sleep deprivation increases Alzheimer's protein. *NIH Research Matters* April 24, 2018.

How Exercise Improves Sleep.
Banno M, Harada Y, Taniguchi M et al. Exercise can improve sleep quality: A systematic review and meta-analysis. *Peer J* 2018;11(6):e5172.

Paper about why writing down your To Do list helps you sleep better.

Scullin MK, Krueger ML, Ballard HK. The effects of bedtime writing on difficulty falling asleep: A polysomnographic study of comparing to-do lists and completed activity lists. *J Exp Psychol Gen* 2018;147(1):139-146.

The Myth of the Eight Hour Sleep.
Hegarty, S. The myth of the eight-hour sleep. *BBC News* February 22, 2012.

Book Suggestion: Why We Sleep by Matthew Walker This is a stellar book that covers many crucial topics about sleep including caffeine intake, jet lag, defining sleep, why sleep is crucial for our health, and why we dream.

Quotes from the book:
"The best bridge between despair and hope is a good night's sleep."

"Sleep is the single most effective thing we can do to reset our brain and body health each day."

Lesson Six: Stockpile Health

Zampieri S, Pietrangelo L, Loefler S et al. Lifelong physical exercise delays age-associated skeletal muscle decline. *J Gerontol A Biol Sci Med Sci* 2015;70(2):163-73.

Handgrip Strength Predicts All-Cause and Premature Mortality.

Kim J. Handgrip strength to predict the risk of all-cause and premature mortality in Korean adults: A 10-year cohort study. *Int J Environ Res Public Health* 2022;19(1):39.

Volpi W, Nazemi R, Fujita S. Muscle tissue changes with aging. *Curr Opin Clin Nutr Metab Care* 2004;7(4):405-10.

Exercise Can Act as a Shield Against Cancer Progression and Metastasis.

Sheinboim D, Parikh S, Manich P et al.

Exercise-induced metabolic shield in distant organs blocks cancer progression and metastatic dissemination. *Cancer Res* 2022;82(22):4164-4178.

Lesson Seven: Staple Your Mouth Shut

Knee replacement surgery does not result in weight loss for overweight or obese patients in the long term.

Pellegrini CA, Song J, Semanik PA et al. Patients less likely to lose weight following a knee replacement: Results from the osteoarthritis initiative. *J Clin Rheumatol* 2017;23(7):355-60.

Messier SP, Gutekunst DJ, Davis C, et al. Weight loss reduces knee-joint loads in overweight and obese older adults with knee osteoarthritis. *Arthritis Rheum* 2005;52(7):2026-32.

World Health Organization's Statistics on Obesity. World Health Organization. Obesity and overweight. June 9, 2021.

Systematic Review of Time-Restricted Feeding on Weight and Other Parameters.

Tsitsou S, Zacharodimos N, Poulia K. Effects of time-restricted feeding and Ramadan fasting on body weight, body composition, glucose responses, and insulin resistance: A systematic review of randomized controlled trials. *Nutrients* 2022;14(22): 4778.

Mind Over Milkshakes Study.
Crum AJ, Corbin WR, Brownell KD et al. Mind over milkshakes: Mindsets, not just nutrients, determine ghrelin response. *Health Psychol* 2011;30(4):424-31.

Book Suggestion: <u>Radical Candor</u> by Kim Scott
This is a business book but I think it perfectly applies to living at our ideal weight. We must admit we have some control over our weight. Scott's concepts of being brutally honest when giving feedback can help us as we seek to live our most vital lives.

Quotes from the book:
"Listen, Challenge, Commit. A strong leader has the humility to listen, the confidence to challenge, and the wisdom to know when to quit arguing and to get on board."

"It's brutally hard to tell people when they are screwing up."

Lesson Eight: Cultivate Closeness

Harvard Study of Adult Development, Longevity and Social Connections
https://www.adultdevelopmentstudy.org/

Social Connection as a Public Health Issue.

Holt-Lunstad J. Social connection as a public health issue: The evidence and a systemic framework for prioritizing the "social" in social determinants of health. *Annu Rev Public Health* 2022;43:193-213.

Hall JA. How many hours does it take to make a friend? *J Social Pers Rela* 2019;36(4):1278-1296.

Lesson Nine: Serving Sparks Hope

Discussion of the Helper's High.
Dossey L. The helper's high. *Explore* 2018;14(6):393-9.

Lower Mortality for Selfless Volunteers.

Konrath S, Fuhrel-Forbis A, Lou A et al. Motives for volunteering are associated with mortality risk in older adults. *Health Psychol* 2012;31(1):87-96.

History of Hotel de Zink.

PaloAltoHistory.org. The Hotel de Zink: A Friend Indeed.

Book Suggestion: <u>Give and Take</u> by Adam Grant
This is an excellent primer on the value of giving and how we can resist our tendency to always consider ourselves first.

Quotes from the book:
"The more I help out, the more successful I become."

"Above all, I want to demonstrate that success doesn't have to come at someone else's expense."

MORE VITALITY RESOURCES

Vitality Explorers

https://www.vitalityexplorers.com/
This is free text message vitality newsletter delivered to your phone once per week.

Vitality Explorer News Podcast

https://vitalityexplorers.substack.com/podcast
This is a weekly podcast about how to enhance your vitality.

Vitality Explorers News on Substack

https://vitalityexplorers.substack.com
This is where Dr. Mishra reviews the world's scientific literature about how to improve your physical, mental, social, and spiritual well-being.

ACKNOWLEDGEMENTS

I t is impossible to properly thank everyone who has helped me produce *Dare To Be Vital*. This second edition represents a complete rewrite with significant additional scientific information and stories. The edition was inspired by my students, patients, and readers of *Vitality Explorer News*. Thank you for reading my material and giving me constructive criticism about how to make it better.

There are dozens of people who have helped me edit the text within these pages. These people have also helped me believe in myself. They have helped me dream greatly, participate in my passions, try something new and most importantly inspire me to help other people with my vitality work and words. I will be forever grateful for their love, support, and expertise.

I'll begin with my wife and daughter, Stephanie and Katie. Stephanie is the beautiful rock upon which this book is built. Katie was my first vitality student and she embraced the ideas embedded here when she was still in high school and helped me edit the first versions.

Patti Davis has been especially helpful during the revising and editing of this second edition. She pushed me to make this better and I can't thank her enough for her coaching, masterful editing skills and patience with my many grammatical errors.

Many others have inspired me to write, revise and publish *Dare To Be Vital.* These people include but are not limited to: Captain Tom Chaby, Giselle Corona, James Cox, David Dvorak, Arielle Eckstut, Steve Elliot, Diane Flynn, Mark Flynn, Paul Gelormini, Jay Gill, Mark Gill, Renata Gomide, Todd Gongwer, Adam Grant, Dr. Jim Hartford, Kevin

Heller, Phil Hellmuth, Dave Keil, Brad Kuish, Jim Levine, John Levin, Chris Loew, Sydney Loew, Ronnie Lott, Anand Mishra, Aneil Mishra, Bec Mitchell, Chris O'Neill, Bill Paull, Dr. William Ranger, Dr. Steve Sampson, Sheryl Sandberg, Jon Sanderson, Charley Scanlyn, Kim Scott, Brent Shaw, Dr. Karen Sutton, Jeff Szorik, Dr. Richard Villar, Dr. Hunter Vincent, Colonel Bill Vivian, Carlos Watson, Tom Whitenight, Dr. Bob Wu, Matt Young, and many others. Many thanks to all of you for helping me #DareToBeVital.

ABOUT THE AUTHOR

D r. Allan Mishra is a board-certified orthopedic surgeon and sports medicine specialist with over 25
years of experience working at the Stanford Medical Center.
He is also a Stanford Continuing Studies Instructor and
leader of the "Energize Your Life" course. Dr. Mishra also
pioneered the use of platelet rich plasma (PRP) for sports
medicine applications and is the founder of *VitalityExplorers.
com*, a movement dedicated to enhancing global vitality.

Dr. Mishra holds BS and MD degrees from the University
of Michigan and completed his orthopedic surgery training
with a fellowship at Stanford in Sports Medicine. Dr. Mishra
has also led vitality discussions and webinars for Apple,
Google, Stanford's Graduate School of Business (GSB), the

University of Michigan, the University of Cambridge, the Campbell Trophy Summit, the Boys and Girls Club of Silicon Valley, and in front of Navy SEALs. Dr. Mishra has also delivered dozens of keynote addresses about regenerative medicine at elite research conferences in the United States, Asia, Europe, and at the United Nations in Geneva. Dr. Mishra has published numerous scientific articles in respected medical journals, and his research has also been featured on the front page of *The New York Times*. He lives in Silicon Valley with his wife, daughter, and awesome dog, Tess.

Made in the USA
Las Vegas, NV
23 February 2023

67995006R00103